The Husbandry of Camelids

The Husbandry of Camelids

Dromedary, Bactrian and Llamoids

Dr. Nityanand Pathak
B.Sc., B.V.Sc. & A.H., M.V.Sc., Ph.D., FNAVSI,
FANA, FMOBS, MAAVN
President, Pashu Chikitski Poshan Avam Kalyan Samiti
113B, Vatika, Sun City Vistaar, Izatnagar-243122, U.P.

Dr. Subodh Kumar Saha
B.V.Sc. & AH, M.Sc.(D), Ph.D.
FNAVS, Post Doc (Australia) Post Doc (USA)
Principal Scientist
Animal Nutrition Division
Indian Veterinary Research Institute
Izatnagar-243122, U.P.

SSPH

SATISH SERIAL PUBLISHING HOUSE
403, Express Tower, Commercial Complex
Azadpur, Delhi-110033 (India)
Phone : 011-27672852, Fax : 91-11-27672046
e-mail : info@satishserial.com, hkjain1975@yahoo.com
Website : www.satishserial.com

Published by :

SATISH SERIAL PUBLISHING HOUSE
403, Express Tower, Commercial Complex, Azadpur, Delhi-110033 (INDIA)
Phone : 011-27672852 Fax : 91-11-27672046
E-mail : info@satishserial.com, hkjain1975@yahoo.com

ISBN 978-93-88020-42-8

Composed, Designed & Printed in India

About the Authors

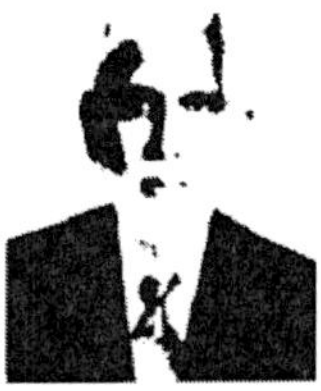

Nityanand Pathak, B.Sc., M.V.Sc, Ph.D, FNAVS, FANA, FMOBS, recipient prize of common wealth Bureaux of Animal Health, England, Jawahar Lal Nehru Award, ICAR, New Delhi, Institute best teacher award, IVRI, Izatnagar, Innovation award of National Research Development Corporation, New Delhi. Scientific contribution include more than 350 research papers, 60 scientific articles, 30 books, 10 compendiums with 350 Co-workers and co-authors. He has also contributed chapters in the books of others countries. He has worked as scientist, project officers, professors, head and director in different institutes. He was buffalo nutrition expert, diplomat and project leader in Buffalo Research Institute, Song Be, Ban Cos, Hochimin City, S. R. Vietnam. Dr. Pathak born on 15th August, 1943 at village Nagwa, District Ballia of Uttar Pradesh, Known as birthplace of Sahid Mangal Pandey, who had been in 1857 revolt against British government.

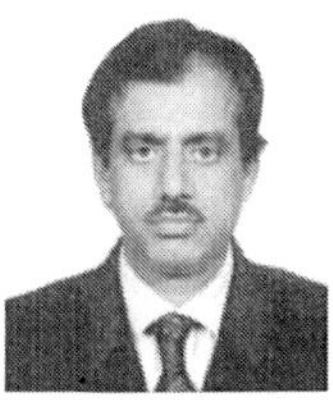

Dr. Subodh Kumar Saha, B.V. Sc. & A.H., M.Sc. (D), Ph.D, FNAVS, Principal Scientist born on 1st November, 1967 in the district of Burdwan, West Bengal and started his career as scientist in the month of August 1995 at Animal Science division, Central Agricultural Research Institute, Port Blair, A & N islands after completion of his management training at National Academy of Agricultural Research Management, Hyderabad. He served as scientist for seven and half years in the Central Agricultural Research Institute at Port Blair, A & N Islands, where he worked on use of alternate feeds in islands for livestock production, use of probiotics for livestock and poultry production, developed different feeding schedule for livestock and poultry, use of tree leaves for goat production. Presently, he is fully engaged in teaching, research and extension activities in Centre of Advanced Faculty Training in Animal Nutrition at Indian Veterinary Research Institute. He is working in the area of unconventional feeds, its detoxification and nutrients utilization for last eight years. Recently, he is working on clinical nutrition to develop a feed based control measure for gastro-intestinal nematodes. He published more than eighty research papers in national and international repute journal. He presented more than 100 conference papers, published many books in animal nutrition, folders, bulletin and monograms. He bagged many awards and recognition in his career like best paper awards from Indian Dairy association, recognition award due to best poster in IVLP work and received fellow from National Academy of Veterinary Sciences due to significant contribution for advancement of veterinary sciences. He has also visited USA and undergone training on **mitigation strategies of methane production** in ruminant livestock at Iowa State University, Ames, Iowa, USA. He also awarded prestigious Endeavour fellowship for post doctorate research in 2015-16 at CSIRO, Brisbane, Australia. He successfully guided more than 20 postgraduate students as an advisor so far.Recently, he visited Berlin, Germany where he presented an invited lecture on scope of unconventional feeds for livestock production in India.

Preface

Camel and llamayads belong to class mammalia, order artiodactyla and suborder tylopoda. The camels are found in Africa and Asia and represented by two genera with one species each. These are *Camelus dromadarius* of tropical hot desert and *Camelus bacterianus* of cold desert. *Camelus bacterianus* is found only in Asian countries. Both species are known as ship of the desert. Llamoids are the native of cold mountains of South America and predominantly found in Peru and Bolivia. These are represented by 4 species comprising of *Llama Glama, L. guanicol,* L. Pacos and *Vicugna vicugna.* The first three species are called Llama or Lama and fourth one Vicugna. The llamas are draught animal and vicugna is soft fibre producing species. Llamoids are not found in any other continent except few members in zoos.

Dromedary camel or single hump camel in Bharat are represented by Bikaneri, Jaisalmeri and Rivarine breeds. The former two breeds are predominantly found in Rajasthan and adjacent parts of the neighboring states *i.e.* Gujarat, Madhya Pradesh and Haryana. Riverine breed is an useful draught camel of river basins and also found along rivers of Uttar Pradesh and west part of Bihar. The population of double humped Camelus bacterianus has reduced to only 100 to 125 animals in Leh area of Bharat in Jammu and Kashmir state. Large number of double humped camels are found in cold desert zone of Central Asia. These are sources of draught, milk, meat, woolen fibre, hide and manure. In Bharat, steps are being taken to protect double humped camels on the farms of state government. Extensive mechanization of transport and spread of network of metalled roads in the desert also the drought utility of dromedary camel has drastically decreased. This is reflected continuously fall in their number. Now at National Research Centre on Camel at Bikaner attempts are being made to transform draught camel to food producing camel such as milk, meat and their nutritious product for human consumption. Camel husbandry is a part of classes of veterinary science in Bharat, Pakistan, Egypt, Israel many countries of north part of America and China. This book has been synthesized to cover syllabi of most of the camel breeding countries.

In preparation of this book we received support of family members that is Sunita-Prafulla Chandra, Priyadarshini-Sanjay, Priyabhashini-Amitabh, Priyambada-Suneel, Rashmi-Ashutosh, Padmashini-Adarsh, Tripti-Ruchin and grand children Ananya, Anshuman, Anubrat, Adya,

Amullya, Atharva, Anavartika and Amyra (of Prof. Pathak) for comfort and tension during the course of work. Sutapa, Akash and Shreyashi (wife, son and daughter of Dr. S.K. Saha) who provided a congenial environment, whole hearted support during the preparation of the manuscript are thankfully acknowledged.

We are also thankful to the publisher Satish Serial Publishing House, New Delhi for publishing this important book for the service of future generation. Lastly authors thanks to all who are directly and indirectly helped for publication of this book successfully.

Dr. Nityanand Pathak
Dr. Subodh Kumar Saha

Contents

About the Authors .... *v*
Preface .... *vii*

1. **Introduction** 1
   - Nomenclature of camelids 2
   - Different camels and cameloids of modern era 3
   - Characteristics of camels and cameloids 6
   - Zoological classification of camelids 8
   - Purpose of camel breeding 8
   - Socio-economic importance of camelids 9
   - Camel – A ship of desert 11
   - World distribution of camelids 12
   - New homes of dromedary 12
   - Temperament of dromedary 14
   - Production potential of camelids 15
   - Future of camelids 19
   - References 19

2. **Haematology of the Camelids** 23
   - Definition of blood 23
   - Composition of blood 23
   - Functions of blood 24
   - Physical properties of blood 24
   - Blood cells 27
   - Erythrocyte count 29
   - Haemoglobin 33
   - Functions of the leucocytes 38
   - Thrombocytes/platelets 38

Blood plasma 39
Blood serum 39
Composition of blood plasma 39
References 47

3. **Digestion and Nutrition** 53
Digestive system of the camelids 53
Functions of the digestive system 64
Factors affecting the digestion 66
Fate of the end products of digestion 67
Feeding behaviour of camel 67
Rumen motility and passage of digesta 71
Rumen contents 74
Rumen microbiology 76
Digestion of feeds and nutrients 77
Rearing of camel calf on milk substitute feeding 79
References 81

4. **Reproduction and Breeding** 87
Male reproductive system 87
Spermatogenesis 94
Spermatozoa 101
The female reproductive system 102
Age at first service 109
Number of service per conception 115
Gestation length / Pregnancy duration 116
Calving interval or Inter-calving period 117
Fertility rate and calving rate 119
Alternate mating system 121
Site of pregnancy 121
Pseudopregnancy 121
Parturition 122

Foetal fluid and membranes 125
Hormonal changes during parturition 126
Post-partum behaviour of the mother 126
Behaviour of the neo-natal calf 127
Breeding season in camelids 127
Sexual behaviour of male camelids 128
Sexual behaviour of female camelids 131
Mating (copulation/coitus) in camels 133
Mating in llamoids 134
Duration of copulation in camelids 134
References 135

5. **The Mammary Glands, Milk and Milk Products** 145
The mammary glands of dromedary 145
Shape and size of the udder and teats of Bactrian camel 148
Let down of milk and milking 149
Colostrum 152
Milk of camelids 154
Composition of milk 155
Milk yield 162
Milk products 169
References 171

6. **Growth in Camelids** 177
Body weight at birth 177
Growth pattern in dromedary camel 182
Growth pattern in Bactrian camel 185
Growth pattern in new world cameloids/llamoids 186
References 186

7. **Meat and Meat Products** 189
Camel veal 190
Camel meat 191

Method of slaughter 191
Body weight of different species at slaughter 191
Carcass characteristics 192
Composition of the dissectable tissues in the carcass 195
Chemical compostion of lean mean 196
Yield of offals and hide 196
Meat of cameloids 197
References 197

8. **Fibre Production** 201
Fibre yield 201
Characteristics of camel hair 203
Characteristics of llamoid wool 204
Hides and skins 205
References 205

9. **Camels for Draught** 209
The riding camels 209
Baggage/draught camels 211
Use of llamoids for riding and work 213
Production of dung energy 213
References 213

10. **Behaviour and Management of the Camel** 215
Behaviour of the one-humped camel 215
Normal values of temperature 216
Respiration rate and pulse (Heart) rate in camelids 216
Camel management practices in the Indian subcontinent 219
References 222

Subject Index 225

Chapter 1

Introduction

The old world camels, the one-humped dromedary (Camelus dromedarius) and double-humped Bactrian (Camelus bactrianus) have been evolved as a source of energy to provide foods and power for mankind in harsh climatic conditions of derserts. Both the species are the sources of milk, meat, fibre and draught power in addition to several useful by-products like hides, fat, faecal pellets and dead carcass for the preparation of feeds for other animals. The two species are widely distributed in the arid and semi-arid areas of Africa and Asia. The dromedaries are mostly found in the hot deserts but also in some parts of cold desert, whereas bactrians are strictly restricted to the cold deserts of central and east Asian countries. Inspite of revolutionary technological developments in the oil and electric operated locomotives, there has been no corresponding decrease in the utility of camels as draught power in their home tracts. Due to their great ability of adaptation in the harsh climatic conditions of deserts, the old world camels are often referred as the 'ship of desert'.

The new world camels, llama (Lama glama), alpaca (L. pacos), guanaco (L. guanaco) and vicuna (Vicugna vicugna)are domesticated and tamed animals except the guanaco which is still wild. These animals are ranched in large flocks on the grasslands at high altitudes for the production of food, fibre and skin. Now-a-days the area of 11 amoids is limited to Peru, Bolivia and some parts of neighbouring states extending north and south of the Andes. The domestic 11 ama is mainly used as a pack animal for carrying 25-30 kg of food products and other commodities to a distance of 15-20 km daily in the mountaineous areas (Flores Ochoa, 1977). The alpaca is primarily bred for fibre production. It produces fine quality wool with little kemp and low felting suitable for the weaving of light weight, soft, smooth and lustrous fabrics.

In India, good breeds of racing and baggage camels have been evolved in the states of 'Thar' desert for riding, force, transport and agricultural operations. The camels are extensively used for pulling the carts, ploughing the fields, pulling persian wheel and buckets for irrigation, carrying 2-4 quintals pack load and riding. A good number of riding camles are employed in different services for travelling through the desert. A considerable number of camels are also kept in the riverine of the Ganga, Gomati and Yamuna in Uttar Pradesh for the haul age of crops from the river basins and also for the transportation of agricultural products to markets. Breeding of camels in these parts is rare because one or two animals are generally kept on stall feeding. The old camels are replaced by new purchases from the annual fairs at Pushkar and other places in Rajasthan and other states.

Although utility of camel in India is still important, little attempt was made in past to organize systematic research for its improvement except the selection followed by the cameleers. Some research projects were completed by the workers at Veterinary College, Bikaner before the establishment of the National Centre for Research on Camels at Bikaner by the Indian Council of Agricultural Research. The main objective of this research centre is to development optimum management practices for maximum utility. A small number of bactrian camels are also found in Laddakh area of India.

Although, exact time of camel existence in India is yet to be traced, it is very new in the sub-continent. Probably camels were introduced in India by the Arabs traders. The presence of camels in India has been referred during the period of king Vikramaditya, when the great poet Kalidas could not pronounce it correctly in Sanskrit landuage in his early days. He called 'utra' in place of the correct word 'ustra', which was instantly corredted by his learned wife Tilottama.

Nomenclature of Camelids

The name of dromedary or one-humped camel has been derived from the Greek word 'dromos' meaning road. Probably this name was given due to the ability of single-humped camel to make their own path in the deserts where human being failed to make in those days. The dromedary camel is also known as Arabian camel probably due to its migration in India from the Arabian countries. The name of double-humped bactrian camel originated from the place 'Bactria' or 'Balka' in the northern region of Afghanistan, although it is neither the place of its origin nor the place of first domestication.

The common names of cameloids viz., llama, alpaca, guanaco and vicuna used by the native Andeans became popular in due course of time. The basis of these names is not known fully.

The zoological nomenclature of the camels and cameloids is based in the basis of morphological differences and breeding performances. Their native names were also used to keep trac with the common names. The consideration of breeding differences vanished later on due to the observations of fertile hybridization between the dromedary and bactrian and between all the four species of 11amoids. Initially the two species of new world cameloids, 11ama and alpaca were included in the genus Camelus of the old world camels, and were named as Camelus glama and Camelus pacos. The remaining two wild varieties, guanaco and vicuna were later also named as Camelus guanaco and Camelus vicugna. The conflict on the nomenclature of camels and cameloids continued and different nomenclatures were suggested for the new world cameloids like Lama, Lacma and Auchenia. The work of Hsu and Benirachke (1967) clearly showed that all the camels and cameloids possess 74 pairs of chromosomes as in the genus Camelus of the old world. Hence, the old and new world camels were ultimately classified into two genera, viz. Camelus for large species and Lama for short cameloids of South America.

Different Camels and Camelolids of Modern Era

The initially recognised three genera of camels of the old and new world, viz. Camelus, Lama and Vicugna were finally classified into two genera merging the latter two of the new world cameloids into genus Lama. The camels are supposed to be evolved from a common ancestor in the North America over a million years ago (Fernandez-Baca, 1978). As stated earlier all the species have 74 pairs of chromosomes (Hsu and Benirschke, 1967, Taylor *et al.*, 1968). The morphological differences are either due to mutation of a single gene or minor re-arrangements of the chromosomes in the changed environment (Taylor *et al.*, 1968). Similarly, old world single and double-humped camels are double-humped in the prenatal life (Denneler de La Tour, 1971). Subsequently one hump developed prominently in those migrated to hot arid region of the Arabian countries and double hump developed in those migrated to the cold-arid regions of central asia (Williams and Payne, 1978). The scarcity of energy in the dry period in hot deserts may be the region for the development of an energy store in the dromedary. The shortage of energy during the winter coupled with high requirement of energy for keeping the body warm might be responsible for the development of double humps in the bactrian camels.

All the camels and cameloids are herbivorous and possess digestion processes similar to that of ruminants. However, these animals have been classified into groups tylopoda due to differences in the morphology of complex stomach, absence of horns and pad like modification of foot. The word 'tylopada' indicates pad like foot structure. At present there are two types of camels in Africa and Asia, and four types of cameloids in the South America.

1. Dromedary or Arabian camel (*Camelus dromedarius*)

It is a long legged tall animal of compact body. The neck is long, narrow and curved, and face is short and triangular being broader at base and narrower towards the blunt oral opening. The ears are short and erect and eyes are small and bright there is no horn. A prominent single hump is present like a contour on the back. The body is covered with short and fine wolly coat. It is a primary source of draught power in the arid and semi-arid areas of the tropical Africa and Asia. Some animals are also found in the temperate climate of Asia. The camels also provide milk, meat and wool in addition to valuable carcass by-products. The dung is used for fuel and manure.

2. Bactrian camel (*Camelus bactrianus*)

Bactrian camels are distinguished from dromedaries on the basis of well developed double hump, dense body coat of long hairs and shorter limbs. The dense body coat provides protection from the frost and cold waves of central asia. The body is massive. It can thrive well on poor pastures and herbages covered under the snow. It is a source of power, milk, meat and wool besides several carcass by-products.

3. Auchenidae or Llamoids or Cameloids

The four species of new world cameloids are called auchenidae as a group. These are much smaller in body size than the old world camels and do not possess any hump. The neck of auchenidae is more or less straight. The hybrids of 4 species are fertile and gradually regress to the original species by third of fourth filial generation. Heterosis due to inter-species crossing is quite apparent. The hybrids of male vicuna and female alpaca, pacovicuma produce finer wool and lighter fleece than their dams. On the other hand hybrids of male 11ama and female alpaca, huarizo produces a thicker and rough fleece than their dams. The utility of huarizo is also unsatisfactory as a pack animal.

The llamas are predominantly found at the high altitude about 4000 to 5500 meters above the sea level in the Andes mountain. In this cold region where temperature ranges from less than zero in night to about 15°C at noon, they thrive well even on very poor herbages like aciachne, agrostis, festucha and muhlembergia. In lean period they also eat some mosses and lichens in an attempt to balance the deficiencies of certain nutrients inadequate in other herbages of low nutritive value. Althouth alpaca may live for few days without water but they prefer to live in the areas of heavy rainfall ensuring adequate water supply and dampness. At present Peru may be considered as the home tract of auchnidae, which was extended to Bolivia and northern region of Argentina. The guanacos are also found in the region of Patagonia and Tierra del Fuego. This species has not yet been domesticated. The vicuna are both wild and domesticated, while the other two species, 11am a and alpaca are domesticated useful animals kept primarily for work and wool production respectively. The wild species are hunted for wool and skin, and meat of all the 4 species is eaten by humans in different forms. Under optimum environment most of the auchenidae attain sexual maturity at about one to two year of ahe (French, 1966, Fernaciez-Baca, 1975).

1. Llama (*Lama glama*)

It is a humpless herbivorous pseudoruminant of about 90-120 kg adult body weight. The animals are reared on the grasslands mainly for the production of fibre and meat besides their use as pack animal. Some milk is also available for human consumption after feeding the calf. Domesticated 11amas are useful for transportation of commodities on the undulating ground of mountaineous regions.

2. Guanaco (*Lama guanaco*)

This species is wild and live on poor grasslands and provide meat and coarse fibres. Adult body weight is about 80 to 90 kg.

3. Alpaca (*Lama pacos*)

A native of Peru and Bolivia, this species is found in wild also. Tamed animals are maintained on ranges for meat and wool production. Adult body weight ranges from 75 to 85 kg.

4. Vicuna (*Lama vicugna* or *Vicugna vicugna*)

This is smallest of the llama species, the adult being 30 to 50 kg of body weight. These are abundant on the Andes mountain area. Like most of the cervidae, an adult male vicuna maintains a 'haram' of 3 to 8 breedable females and their progeny. Earlier it was classified as a separate genus, Vicugna.

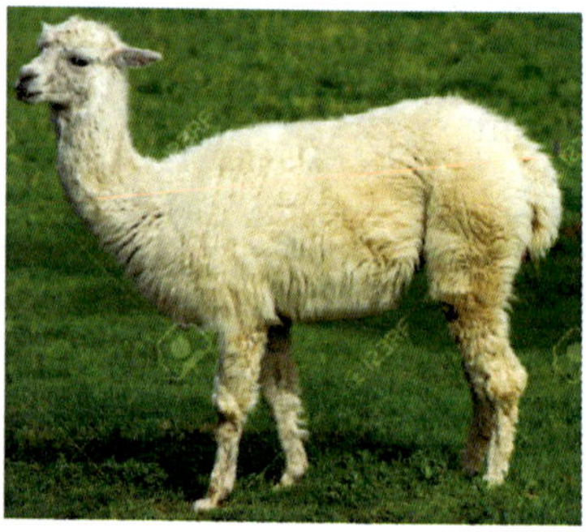

Vicugna (*Lama vicugna*)

Characteristics of Camels and Cameloids

The camels are intermediary to top feeders or browsers depending on the herbage available, and had better developed sensory organs for the selective feeding of more succulent and less fibrous feeds. Indeed they are capable to thrive exclusively on rough fibrous feeds of low nutritional quality, because high retention time of feeds in the gastro-intestinal tract provides longer period for the microbial digestion of cellulosic material and protein synthesis from the recycled nitrogen (Heller *et al.*, 1986, Lechner-Doll, 1986). The bifid upper lip and scoop shaped longer lower lip are highly mobile. These are coupled with upper incisors provide special skill of shorting out edible parts even from the thorny shrubs and trees, and long neck is helpful in browsing on tall trees. Some observations also indicate that the camel (Dromedary) prefers grasses and selective while alpaca prefers browsing but also less selective (McDowell, 1986). The author has observed both, grazing on small herbs and browsing on shrubs, trees and bamboo in the camels of the Gangetic revine. They browse on neem (*Azadirachta indica*), peepal (*Ficus religiosa*), gular (*Ficus lecor*), beri (*Zizyphus* spp.), bamboos , babul (*Acacis nilotica*) and many other plants found in the area.

The protein utilization efficiency is more efficient and camels are capable to meet their requirement through higher recycling of nitrogen, which may be 90-96 per cent in the camels and llamas during the feeding of low protein diets (Ali *et al.*, 1977, Hinderer, 1978, Engelhardt, 1978, Mousa *et al.*, 1983). The rate of urea degradation in the forestomach of camelids depends on dietary protein content. On the feeding of a diet containing about 6 per cent crude protein in dry matter, the urea degradation was about 86 per cent, which significantly fell down to 74 per cent on feeding of 9.6 per cent crude protein in ration and 47 per cent on feeding of 13 per cent crude protein in ration on dry matter basis. A considerable rise in the level of plasma urea occurs due to feeding of high protein rations, although there is significant decrease in the degradation of urea (Emmanuel *et al.*, 1976).

The large size of camel appearing disadvantageous is actually useful because it takes longer time to heat up the body exposed to direct solar radiation. Thus, helps in the maintenance of tolerable body temperature for longer period and enables camels to travel long distance in deserts for searching food and water. The heavy hump stores a large amount of fat living rest of the body almost free from the subcutaneous layer of adipose tissue. This facilitates more efficient dissipation of body heat (Cloudsley-Thompson, 1969). In favourable feeding condition, a full formed hump is about 20 per cent of the body weight (Emmanuel, 1981). The hump fat is mobilized for the supply of energy requirement of the body during the scarcity. The long, slender and thin limbs with large foot are very useful for walking across the sandy deserts. Wide and flat digital bones are present embedded in a broad cutaneous pad forming the sole of the foot. The foot pads expand with the pressure of body when put on the ground. This facilitates movement in the sand. Thickly cornified sole and pads on the chest and all the four legs keep the body of camel elevated from the hot sandy surface while sitting. Arched abdominal aspect is also helpful in elevating the body from the ground in sitting posture. The horny layer is less sensitive and enables the camels to tread across the desert in hot sun. A riding camel can trot at a speed of 5-6 km per hour and fast run at a speed of 6-12 km per hour (Gillespie, 1962). Bactrian camels are normally ridden a distance of 50-70 km and carry pack loads for 30-40 km a day (Knoess, 1977, Chapman, 1985).

The external nares are almost horizontal and close to each other in front. The presence of a thick layer of hairs in the nostrils prevent the entrance of sand during breathing in whirls and storms. Similarly, long eye lashes and a well-developed third eyelid or nictitating membrane provide protection to the eyes against foreign bodies including sand and dust.

The body is covered with soft, fine and dense woolly hairs during the winter for protection from the cold. These are shed off gradually during the hot season for facilitating the dissipation of body heat. The woolly coat is longer and denser in bactrian and 11amas, because they live in the colder regions.

Zoological Classification of Camelids

The widely accepted zoological classification of camelidae (Honacki *et al.*, 1982) in animal kingdom is as follows:

Kingdom	Animalia	
Phylum	Cordata	
Class	Mammalia	
Subclass	Ungulata	
Order	Artiodactyla	
Suborder	Tylopoda	
Familae	Camelidae	
Genus	(1) Camelus and	(2) Lama
Species	*Camelus bactrianus*	*Lama glama*
	C. dromedarius	*L. pacos*
		L. guanaco
		Vicugna vicugna

Purpose of camel breeding

The old world camels are main sources of draught power in the arid and semi-arid regions of Africa and Asia. The dromedaries are primarily adapted to the harsh dry climatic conditions extending from Sahara in Africa to Thar in India. Dromedaries can go without water for several days, can walk on sand more than 20 km a day and can thrive on the scanty grasses and thorny bushes containing low amount of protein and easily digestible energy. They are used for riding, carrying pack loads upto 400kg, ploughing, pulling cart and persian wheel, crushing sugarcane and rotating oil extraction mills. The bactrians are used for almost similar agro-industrial operations in the cold deserts of central Asia. They are capable of walking on snow and can dig herbages under snow for feeding. Light weight, slender camels of both species are used for riding due to their faster pace in arid areas. In addition to draught power, they also provide nutritious milk and meat for humans. Both dromedary and bactrian camels are good yielders and may produce 1000 to 3000 litres of milk during a lactation period of 250 to 400 days. The milk contains 5-6 per cent fat and also high levels of protein and milk sugar (Kulaeva, 1964, Ohri and Joshi, 1961, Sohail, 1983, Meredov,1984). Recently an organized dairy of dromedary has been started near Riyadh in Saudi Arabia during 1985. The milk is supplied in packed cartons after pasteurization and homogenization. Fine wool is used for the preparation of garments while coarse wool is used for carpet making.

The new world cameloids, llama, alpaca, guanaco and vicuna are primarily reared on natural herbages for the production of meat and wool. Some milk is also available for human consumption from the domesticated flocks. Large species are used for transportation and haulage. Wool and hairs are used for the manufacture of fine fabrics, rugs, carpets and ropes.

All species of camels and llamas provide large quantity of hides and skins for industrial uses, and bones and dung for manure production. A small amount of dung is also used as fuel.

Socio-Economic Importance of Camelids

In their home tracts, the camels and llamas are usually reared on pastures by the nomads and tribes. The number of camel shows the economic strength of a family which determines the social status. In several African and Arabian countries man dependence on camel is more in comparison to other domestic animals and agricultural crops. The afro-arabian pastoralists have been formally categorized into three classes, viz., (i) The Murrah Bodouin community of Arabia is almost entirely dependent on their camels for earning their livelihood. Due to this reason they care their camels more than the any other group; (ii) In the Gabra community of Kenya and Afar community of Etheopia, camels are the main component of mixed animal husbandry. They raise considerable number of sheep and goats alongwith camels. In this system dependence is distributed on different livestock and people feel more secure against the calamities; (iii) The Kababish arabs of Sudan and the Jawabis of Egypt live in organised villages and also cultivate grains (Cole, 1975).

Free living lifestyle coupled with straight forward behavior, simple living and limited requirements are the characteristics of nomads and tribals. People of these communities dislike any type of unusual authority to control their routine activity. Indeed, they have their social culture developed to cater the requirement of security and peaceful coexistence. For this purpose each community has its head and a group of elders for guiding and keeping the community in order. Pastoralist nomads move together in groups along with their livestock. This practice has been evolved for protection against disasters and insecurity. Earlier there was no defined territorial limits in the pastoralist tribes but now it is developing with the colonisation in many countries. There is frequent occurance of drought in the deserts and camels are most suitable for the shifting of families and households to places near the water resources.

In the nomads and tribes, animals and animals products are the main capital which are used for the payment of compensation against injuries and losses, for dowry and gift to young ones for establishing their own herds for earning livelihood. After marriage, couple wishes to establish their own household and for this purpose their parents gift them animals as per their capacity depending on the number of camels and other livestock and the number of dependents expected to part away after marriage. Although, there is considerations for the women and female childs but as usual like settled societies in nomads and tribes also male dominance and preference for male child are quite visible. In most of the cases, the females are rated half of the males value, e.g., in Somalia for a serious injury to a man, a fine of 100 camels is imposed, whereas for similar injury to a woman the fine is only 50 camels. For the purpose of exchange one camel is equal to nine sheep (Mares, 1954).

In the Gabbra, Rendille and Somali communities, division of labour among the family members is defined and work responsibility depends on age, sex and physical strength. The ladies are mostly involved in house jobs and management of the livestock left at home for milk. The animals are grouped according to species, age and milk production and herded/flocked in the temporary enclosures made of thorny bushes for providing protection against predators and animal lifters (Torry, 1971, Dahl and Hjort, 1979, Hartley, 1979). The Kababish families follow another system of herding camels. By routine 3 or 4 men from a group of families are given the responsibility of camel herd management. They collect 100-150 camels and may stay away with them for several days in search of fodder and water. The goats are kept near the camps (Asad, 1970).

The social organization in camel breeding communities of India is some what different. In Rajsthan, although herds of camels alongwith sheep flock, goats and cattle together or separate are moved to long distances for feeding during scarcity, but all have settled homes and return back with the normalization of the conditions following the rains. While out with their livestock, they earn their livelihood through the sale of milk and ghee, and rent in the form of cash or food grains for herding the livestock in fields for manuring. Animal exchange system is now-a-days very rare. There are well-organised markets and fairs for the sale and purchase of livestock. Animal fairs of Pushkar in Rajsthan, Bateshwar and Gobindshah in Uttar Pradesh are famous for the sale and purchase of camels besides other livestock. In India, mostly there is joint family system and parentral properties are automatically transferred to the succesors, mostly the males. Recent changes in laws have now provided rights to female children also.

With the exposure of nomads and tribes to modern developments, a significant change in their life style may be observed all over the world. This is further helped by the international organisations involved in human welfare. Now most of the nomads and tribes are adopting to permanent settlement in villages and towns and organising systematic animal and crop husbandry practices. They are also being educated for developing cottage industries utilizing their own raw materials for more remunerative returns.

Camel – A Ship of Desert

The term is normally used for the dromedaries, which are capable to thrive and work in the different conditions of the dry-hot deserts of Sahara, Arab and Thar. Camel caravans may walk upto 40 km a day, loaded with 150-200 kg goods on the sand where it is very difficult to make roads and rail routes (Knoess, 1977). In India, the camels are used to carry pack load of about 300 kg for 15-20 km daily. They are also used for ploughing, pulling Persian wheels for irrigation and pulling carts. Camels are the main source of transportation of commodities from the sandy areas to towns and vice-versa. The term 'ship of desert' may also be applicable to the bactrian camels which easily carry loads and ridden on the snow covered 1 and in their home tract.

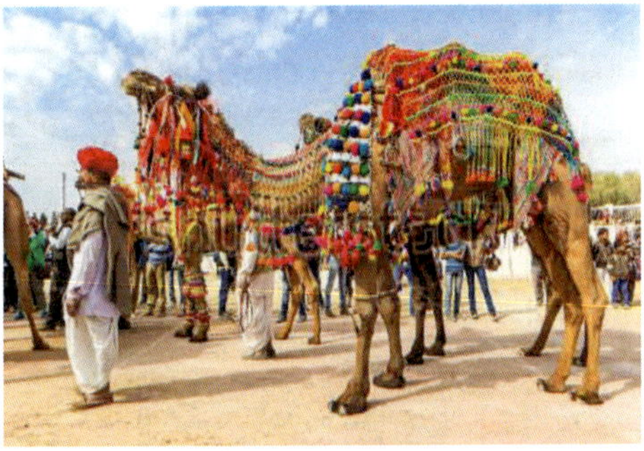

Decorated Camel
(*Courtsey:* Pushkar mela, Rajasthan)

World distribution of Camelids

The dromedary and bactrian camels are widely distributed through out hot and cold deserts and also in riverines of some tropical countries of Africa and Asia. In Africa, only single-humped camels are found, whereas in Asia both single-humped and double-humped and their hybrids are prevalent. Both these species are domesticated animals except some small herds of feral dromedary in the National Parks of Africa and one or two small herds of wild bactrian in the Gobi desert of central Asia. The llamoids are restricted to the Andean mountain and adjoining hilly areas, and their number may be about one million. The distribution and growth pattern of camelids as presented by FAO (1990) are shown in Table 1.

New homes of dromedary

Sometimes in the past small herds of dromedary were introduced in the tropical regions of North America and western part of Australia, and feral herds are still found in these areas. A few herds of dromedary have been domesticated in the South Africa mainly for draught purpose in difficult areas. The camels in their new homes are performing satisfactorily and their herds are being maintained without any problem.

Table 1. Distribution of camels (FAO, 1990) in thousands.

Continent/Country	1979-81	1988	1990
World	16691	19099	19450
Africa	12400	14288	14600
Burundi	6	5	5
Chad	432	517	540
Djibouti	51	58	59
Egypt	91	178	190
Ethiopia	980	1060	1080
Kenya	608	790	810
Libya	134	185	193
Mali	230	231	241
Mauritania	734	810	820
Morocco	157	36	43
Niger	404	417	420
Nigeria	17	18	18

Senegal	7	15	15
Somalia	5533	6841	6855
Sudan	2611	2732	2800
Tunisia	173	184	187
ASIA	4051	4511	4641
Afghanistan	267	265	265
Bahrain	1	1	1
China	597	475	475
Gaza strip	1	1	1
India	1050	1390	1450
Iran I R	29	27	27
Iraq	72	55	59
Israel	11	10	10
Jordon	13	18	15
Kuwait	5	8	6
Mongolia	601	547	560
Oman	41	82	87
Pakistan	844	957	990
Qatar	10	21	24
Saudi Arabia	277	405	405
Syria	7	4	5
Turkey	12	3	3
United Arab Em.	57	99	115
Yemen	158	144	144
USSR/Central Asia	235	300	300

Temperament of dromedary

Apparently dromedaries appear indifferent to surroundings and one may observe that they do not care for the horns of vehicles and presence of other domestic animals. However, there are many folk lores about the revengeful nature of the camels. They carry any wrong done to them for long time and punish the culprit when get an opportunity. An enraged camel is very dangerous and may bite the owner or anyone teasing him or forcing him to work or drive. The camels have great affinity for their native place and often sold camels return back to their native place travelling long distance (Dickson, 1951).

Table 2: Details of camels by age and sex in rural and urban combined (19th Livestock census in 2012)

S.No.	State/ UT	Male			Female			Total Camel
		Under 4 Years	4 Years and Above	Total	Under 4 Years	4 Years and Above	Total	
	(1)	(2)	(3)	(4)	(5)	(6)	(7)	(8)
1	Andaman & Nicobar Islands	0	0	0	0	0	0	0
2	Andhra Pradesh	30	40	70	54	30	84	154
3	Arunachal Pradesh	3	0	3	19	23	42	45
4	Assam	252	255	507	211	8	219	726
5	Bihar	3640	4900	8540	175	144	319	8859
6	Chandigarh	0	0	0	0	0	0	0
7	Chhattisgarh	34	591	625	18	2	20	645
8	Dadra & Nagar Haveli	0	0	0	0	0	0	0
9	Daman & Diu	0	0	0	0	0	0	0
10	Goa	0	1	1	0	0	0	1
11	Gujarat	3710	13181	16891	4342	9182	13524	30415
12	Haryana	993	4609	5602	1868	11375	13243	18845
13	Himachal Pradesh	104	53	157	17	3	20	177
14	Jammu & Kashmir	151	652	803	17	105	122	925
IS	Jharkhand	0	2	2	0	1	1	3
16	Karnataka	52	75	127	9	15	24	151
17	Kerala	2	0	2	3	1	4	6
18	Lakshadweep	0	0	0	0	0	0	0
19	Madhya Pradesh	763	960	1723	553	1146	1699	3422
20	Maharashtra	35	87	122	20	40	60	182
21	Manipur	0	0	0	0	0	0	0
22	Meghalaya	7	0	7	0	0	0	7
23	Mizoram	0	0	0	0	0	0	0
24	Nagaland	36	56	92	0	0	0	92
25	NCT of Delhi	74	25	99	28	30	58	157
26	Odisha	349	471	820	8	7	15	835
27	Puducherry	0	0	0	0	0	0	0
28	Punjab	139	256	395	74	224	298	693
29	Rajasthan	43564	103881	147445	48025	130243	178268	325713
30	Sikkim	0	0	0	0	0	0	0
31	Tamil Nadu	6	8	14	1	4	5	19
32	Tripura	0	0	0	0	0	0	0
33	Uttar Pradesh	2328	4044	6372	671	892	1563	7935
34	Uttarakhand	0	0	0	0	0	0	0
35	West Bengal	99	149	248	4	15	19	267
Total		56371	134296	190667	56117	153490	209607	400274

Production potential of camelids

In addition to their common uses for riding and draught, the various camelid species are also reared for the production of milk, meat and wool. The important by-products are hides, skins and dung. Old world camels, dromedary and bactrian are good milk yielders and spare 5 to 10 litres milk daily for human consumption after nursing their calves. Weaning can be practiced safely at 6-7 months without hampering the lactation of dams. The cameloids of new world are better sources of good quality fibre (wool). Considerable amount of camel dung is used as fuel for domestic purposes. The various production functions of camelids are briefly described.

1. Milk production : Probably there is no precise breeding programme for milk production, but random selection practices have increased the inherent milk production potential significantly. Average milk production per lactation ranges from about 1000 litres to more than 400 litres during the lactation period of 10-18 months in dromedaries. The milk production is significantly influenced by the parity, size of animal, climate and nutritional supply (Leese, 1927, Yasin and Wahid, 1957, Iwema, 1960, Sharma and Bhargava, 1963, Lakosa and Shokin, 1964, Rao *et al.*, 1970, Dahl and Hjort, 1976, knoess, 1977, Sohail, 1983, Meredov, 1984). The correct estimation of milk yield under pastoral management is very difficult because milking frequency is highly variable. It ranges from once daily to even more than six times daily in different pastoral communities of Africa (Bremaud, 1969, Spenser, 1973, Cole, 1975, Knoess, 1977). Indian hot desert camels are milked twice daily at about 12 hour interval and occasionally 3 or 4 times a day.

The milk yield in bactrian camels is 700 to 2000 litres during the lactation period of 12-18 months (Terent jev, 1963, Kulaeva, 1964, Chapman, 1985). Some rare specimen may yield as high as 5000 litres milk in a lactation period of about 2 years (Williamson and Payne, 1978). The peak lactation reaches during the third month of lactation (Kulaeva, 1964, Cherepenova, 1986). In Kazakhstan, camel farms of 100-120 animals are quite prevalent but for economic dairy farming a herd of 1500-2000 animals has been suggested (Dshakupov and Abdrakhimov, 1986).

The hybrids of dromedary X bactrian produce more milk (B1agovescenskii, 1963) which may be about 25 per cent higher than the average of the parents (Dzhumagulov, 1983).

Being much smaller in body size than the old world camels, the 11amoids produce small amount of milk for human uses. The milk left after suckling the cria is 40 to 1200 ml daily in alpaca. The milk is white in colour and more sweet than the milk of cow (Jimenez O choa, 1970).

2. Meat production : The new world cameloids were hunted for meat, fibre (wool) and skin in the Andes hills and surrounding areas in South America. In 1963, there were about 2.8 million alpacas in Peru. The body weight at slaughter ranges from 57 to 72 kg (average 67 kg) for the males and 55 to 66 kg (average 59 kg) for the females; and carcass weights were 32 and 30 kg for the two sexes respectively. The average carcass yield has been reported to be about 39 per cent. The meat of alpaca has high protein and low fat percentage (Tapia Cano, 1965). Now attempts are being made to rear vicuna for meat and wool production by the Peruvian Forest Service (Anonymous, 1966). Earlier vicuna were distributed in Chile, Argentina, Bolivia, Peru and Ecuador. Now they are reported to be extinct in Ecuador and probably in Argentina also (Jungius, 1972). The adult body weight of 11ama, alpaca and vicuna is about 120, 70 and 40 kg respectively. The carcass yield of alpaca under well finished condition is about 60 per cent in males and 55 per cent in females (Fernandez-Baca, 1975).

The double-humped camels of Central Asia are the heavy animals and males may attain more than 800 kg body weight at maturity. Carcass yield varies from less than 50 per cent in poor old animals to more than 60 per cent dressed carcass in well finished young animals (Terent jev, 1963, Kulaeva, 1964, Cerenpuncag and Davaa, 1967. Percentage of fatty tissue is higher in castrated males than the carcasses of females (Zhang *et al.* 1983). The meat is consumed as normal cooked local products and also processed for the preparation of sausages and other preserved products for consumption at later occasions or for carrying to distant places without spoilage.

The use of dromedary for meat production is rather recent except in a few countries of Africa where camel meat is traditionally eaten during the scarcity caused by recurring droughts. The animals are slaughtered indiscriminately without the consideration of age and sex. Carcass yield ranges from 45 to 63 per cent and like other species dressing percentage depends on the nutritional status of the animals. Hump fat is more in aged than in the young camels (Wilson, 1978, Sohail, 1983, Babiker, 1984). The carcasses are often graded into three grades on the basis of muscle, fat and bone percentage. The percentage of lean meat is highest and fat is medium in grade 1 carcass, whereas lean meat percentage is lowest and fatty tissues and depot fats are almost absent in grade 3 carcasses. Largest proportion of carcasses fall in grade 2 containing less lean meat and more fatty tissue than the grade 1 carcasses (Kuznetsov and Tret'yakov, 1970). The meat production potential of bactrian camels is more than the dromedaries, and former can compete with the beef cattle of that area in performance (Aueljbekov, 1967).

Interspecies and intraspecies cross-breeding improves the productivity of hybrids. The hybrids of dromedary and bactrian camels are larger and produce more meat and milk than either of the parents (Blagovescenskii, 1963, Kulaeva, 1964).

The blood of camel is also consumed by some nomadic communities of Africa, About 5-6 litres blood may be bled two times every month from the optimally fed Turkana camels (Pratt and Gwynne, 1977).

3. Fibre (wool) Production : Both wool and hairs are produced by all camelidae. The growth of hair coat is more in cold than the hot climate. The quality of wool is significantly affected by the sex, age, nutrition and environmental temperature. Annual fibre clip in the new world cameloids (11amas) is 1-4 kg in different species (Fernandez-Baca, 1975). The quality of wool is quite good in small species. Average fibre diameter ranges from 13.44 to 19.68 m in the vicuna, guanaco and 11ama being coarser in 11ama. It compares in quality with cashmere fibre with diameter range of 14.73 to 15.50 m and Turkish gairy goat fibre of 17.63 m average diameter (Utkanlar *et al.*, 1963).

Annual hair yield in bactrian camels is 2.8 to 18 kg and fieece contains about 20-27 per cent coarse fibres. The yield of wool is significantly influenced by the age, sex, pregnancy and lactation (Kulaeva, 1964, Cerenpuncag and Davaa, 1967, Luvsan, 1969, Chapman, 1985).

The wool of dromedary is light and durable. It is good for making blankets and woolen fabrics. The dromedaries of hot zone yield half to 1.5 kg wool annually (Nanda, 1957, Singh, 1966, Hartley, 1979, Sohail, 1983). The dromedaries of cold region compete well with the bactrians in wool production and may produce upto 12 kg wool per year (Terentjev, 1963). The hair of mane also provides materials for the industrial uses. Tail hair is quite rough and mostly used for rope making.

4. Hide production : The hide of camelidae is considered to be of inferior quality. Larger proportion of hides and skins are used locally for the preparation of water bags and tents. The yield of hide is quite variable and in dromedaries it is 27 to 39 kg per animal (Terentjev, 1963). The skin of old world camel is much thicker than the cattle and its processing yields poor quality leather.

The skin of new world 11amoids is priced product due to its extensive use in the preparation of warm garments for babies and fancy items for the ladies as well as decoration items for household uses.

5. Draught power : The camels are well known for beast of burden and probably they are only animals capable to work on sands, which justifies the synonym 'ship of desert' used for the dromedaries as well as bactrian camels. The bactrians are the main draught animals of the Gobi desert and other parts of central asia.

The members of auchenidae are used for riding and carrying pack loads in the Andes hill regions and other parts of the South America.

The dromedaries are used for riding, pulling the carts, drawing of Persian wheels for watering, ploughing the field and operating sugarcane crushers and oil extracting mills (Matharu, 1966). Normally dromedaries are used single and rarely in pairs. Occasionally they are also used in a team with the bullock or working buffalo (Leese, 1927).

The Indian draught camels are capable to plough at a pace of 2-3 km per hour. The working hours should be 3-4 hours in early morning and if necessary, 2-3 hours in late evening. Total working hours should be restricted to 5-6 hours daily. In traditional local carts they are capable to pull a load of 300-400 kg which may be doubled by using improved carts (Singh, 1963). Recently much advancements have been made in designing the pneumatic carts with wheels fitted on ball-bearings. Such carts are pulled by one or two camels depending on the size and these may have one or two pairs of tyres. Now-a-days two types of such camel carts, one for carrying the goods and another fitted with seats for passengers are commonly seen in most parts of the Indian deserts. The Ethiopean and Sudanese camels carry 300-400 kg pack loads in four sacks and can plough 1 hectare 1 and in 12-20 hours depending on the depth of furrows (Knoess, 1977).

The bactrian camels are as well used as saddle animals and for draught purposes. The baggage carriers may cover 4 to 4.5 km per hour (Terentjav, 1963, Cerenpuncag and Davaa, 1967). The hybrids of dromedary and bactrian are generally more sturdy than pure bred parents.

Among the new world cameloids, the 11amas and guanacos are preferred for draught and riding purposes. Unlike old world camels, the hybrids of 11ama and alpaca known as Huarizo is a bad pack animal. The 11amoids are very notorious animals and do not hesitate spitting on the face of the rider when tired. On packing heavier loads they lie down and do not respond unless the load is reduced to their carrying capacity.

Future of camelids

Inspite of the development of mechanical, chemical and electrical operated transports, the camelids will continue to serve the mankind still in many countries as a beast of burden. The uses of camelids are now been diverted more for the production of meat, milk, wool and also fur and pelt from the young ones preferably from the soft skin 11amoids. In recent past, demand of fancy items of 11amoid skin has increased and now it has increased demand in international markets. In many countries breeding policies have been modified to make the camelids main sources of meat and milk besides as usual use of wool producers.

References

Asad, T. 1970. The Kababish Arabs : Power, authority and consent in a nomadic tribe. C. Hurst and Co., London.

Aue ljbekov, K. 1967. Camel breeding-a profitable field. Konevod. Konnyi Sport, 5:6.

Babiker, M.M. 1984. Abundance and economic potential of camels in Sudan. J. Arid Environ., 7: 377.

Blago vescenskii, V. 1963. Reserves in the production of milk and meat. Konevod. Konnyi Sport, 33: 8.

Bremaud, O. 1969. Trans ILCA- Notes on camel production in the northern districts of the Republic of Kenya. IEMVT, 105.

Cerepuncag, S. And Davaa, R. 1967. Camel breeding in Mongolia. Mezhdunar sel'khoz Zh., 11: 107.

Chapman, M.J. 1985. Mongolia : Bactrian camels. World Anim. Rev., No. 55: 14.

Cherepenova, V.P., Musaev, Z.M. and Belokobylenko, V.T. 1986. The chemical composition of camel milk. Zhivotnovodstvo, 3: 55.

Cloudslay-Thompston, J.L. 1969. Camel. Encyclopedia Americana, 5: 261.

Cole, D.P. 1975. Nomads of the nomads: The Al Murrah Bedouin of the Empty Quarter. P. 179. Aldine Pub. Co. , Chicago, USA.

Dahl, G. and Hjort, A. 1976. Having herds: Pastoral herd growth and household economy. Department of Anthropology, University of Stockholm, Sweden.

Dennler De La Tour, D. 1971. Inheritance of the hump in the camel, dromedary and camel X dromedary cross. Anim. Breed. Abstr.

Dickson, W.M. 1951. Endocrine glands. In: Duke's Physiology of Domestic Animals. Cornell University Press, London.

Dzhakupov, T.D. and Abdrakhimov, A.O. 1986. Development of camel husbandry in Kazakhstan. Zhivotnovodstvo, 6: 14.

Dzhumagulov, I.K. 1083. Hybridization in camel breeding. Zhivotnovodstvo, 9: 46

Emmanuel, B. 1981. Fatty acid synthesis in camel (Camelus dromed-arius) hump and sheep (oris aries) tail fat. Comp. Biochem. Physiol., 68B: 551.

Emmanuel, B., Howard, B.R. and Emady , M. 1976. Urea degradation in the camel. Canadian J. Anim. Sci., 56: 595.

Engelhardt, W. von 1978. Adaptation to low protein diets in some mammals. Proc. Zodiac Symp. Adapt. Centre Agric. Pub. Document, Washington.

FAO. 1990. Production year book, FAO, Rome.

French, M.H. 1966. The Auchenidae. World Rev. Anim. Prod. 2(3): 89.

Fernandez-Baca, S. 1975. Alpaca raising in the high Andes. World Anim. Rev. No. 14: 1.

Fernandez-Baca, S. 1978. Llamoids or New World Camelidae. In: An Introduction to Animal husbandry in Tropics. 3rd ed. Longman, London.

Gillespie, I.A. 1962. Riding camels of the Sudan. Sudan J. Vet. Sci. Anim. Husb., 3: 37.

Hartley, B.J. 1979. The dromedary of the horn of Africa. Proc. Workshop on camels, Khartoum, Sudan.

Heller, R., Lechner, M. and Engelhardt, W.V. 1986. Forestomach motility in the camel (Camelus dromedarius). Comp. Biochem. Physiol., 84A: 285.

Iwema, S. 1960. The ship of desert. Veeteelt-en Zuivelberichten, 3: 390.

Jimenez Ochoa, R. 1970. Some aspects of alpaca milk. Tropicales y de Altura, Peru No. 4: 60.

Jungius, H. 1972. Bolivia and the vicuna. Oryx, 11: 335.

Knoess, K.H. 1977. The camel as a meat and milk animal. World Animal Rev. No. 22: 139.

Kulaeva, V. 1964. The production of the bactrian camel. Konevod. Konnyi Sport, 34: 9.

Kuznetsov, V.A. and Tretyakov, V.N. 1970. Carcass classification in the Turkmen single-humped camel. Trudy Turk. Sel'Khoz., 15: 130.

Lakosa, I.I. and Shokin, V.A. 1964. Milk production in camel. Sci. Tech. Agric. Pub., Kolos, Moscow.

Lechner-Doll

Leese, A.S. 1927. A treatise on the one-humped camel in health and disease. Haynes and Sons, Stamford.

Luvsan, B. 1969. Some economic and biological traits of Mongolian two-humped camels. Anim. Breed. Abst. (1972), 40: 570.

Mares, R.G. 1954. Animal husbandry, animal industry and animal diseases in the Somalil and Protectorate. Part I and II. British Vet. J., 110: 411-470.

Matharu, B.S. 1966. Camel care. Indian Farming, 16(7): 19.

McDowell, R.E 1986. Improvement of livestock production in warm climate. W.H. Freeman and Co., San Francisco.

Meredov, B. 1984. Some problems of camel breeding in Turkmenia. Konevod. Konnyi Sport, 12: 22.

Mousa, H.M. , Ali, K.G. and Hume, I.D. 1983. Effects of water deprivation on urea metabolism in camels, desert sheep and desert goats fed dry desert grass. Comp. Bio Chem. Phy Siol., 74A: 715.

Muller, 1982.

Nanda, P.N. 1957. Camels and their Management. Indian Council of Agricultural Research, New Delhi.

Ohri, S.P. and Joshi, B.K. 1961. Composition of milk of camel. Indian vet. J., 38: 514.

Pratt, D.J. and Gwynne, M.D. 1977. Range 1 and Management and Ecology in East Africa. Hodder and Stoughton, London.

Rao, M.B., Gupta, R.G. and Dastur, N.N. 1970. Camel's milk and milk products. Indian J. Dairy Sci., 23: 71.

Sharma, V. D. and Bhargava, K.K. 1963. The Bikaneri camel. Indian Vet. J., 40: 639.

Singh, H. 1963. Handbook of Animal husbandry for extension workers. Ministry of Food and Agric., New Delhi.

Singh, H. 1966. Camel care. Intensive Agric., January, 9.

Sohail, M.A. 1983. The role of the Arabian camel (Camelus dromedarius) in animal production. World Rev. Anim. Prod., 19: 37.

Spencer, P. 1973. Nomads in alliance: Symbiosis and growth amont the Rendille and Samburu of Kenya. Oxford University Press, London.

Tapia Cano, C. 1965. Production of alpaca meat. Vida Agric., 42: 499.

Taylor, K.M., Hungerford, D.A., Snyder, R.L. and Ulmer, F.A.Jr.1968. Uniformity of karyotypes in the camelidae. Cytogenetics, 7: 7.

Terentjev, S.M. 1963. Camel breeding in Astrakhan Province. Zivotnovodstvo, 25: 54.

Torry, W.I. 1971. Animal husbandry and social organization among the Gabbra, with notes on the Rendille tribes. In: Rangel and management and ecology in East Africa. Hodder and Stoughton, London (1977).

Utkanlar, N., Imeryuz, F., Oznacar, K. and Muftuoglu, S. 1963. Studies on the fineness and colour characteristics of the Turkish hairy goat wool and their comparison with those of Cashmere, 11ama, vicuna and guanaco wools. Lalhan Zootek. Arast. Enst. Derg., 3(2): 8.

Williamson, G. and Payne, W.J.A. 1978. An introduction to Animal Husbandry in the Tropics. 3rd ed. Longman, London.

Wilsdn, R.T. 1978. Studies on the livestock of southern Darfur, Sudan. V. Notes on camels. Tropical Anim. H1th. Prod., 10: 19.

□□□

Chapter 2

Haematology of the Camelids

Definition of Blood

The blood, a complex fluid-solid system, is a connective tissue. Although, itself contained in the cardiovascular system, it has close connection with almost all body cells. The blood is formed of corpuscles or cells and other particles suspended in the plasma. The plasma is a colloidal medium. On the following grounds blood may be classified as connective tissue :

1. The origin of blood is mesoderm.
2. The blood connects almost all functional component of the body.
3. The fluid or colloidal part of the blood predominates.
4. Many of the blood cells originate from the reticulo-endothelial system.
5. Some of the blood cells can undergo mutation.

Composition of Blood

The blood is made of a colloidal medium known as plasma and three types of corpuscles or cells suspended in the plasma. The cells are erythrocytes or red blood cells (RBC), leucocytes or white blood cells (WBC) and thrombocytes or platelets. The following flow chart gives information about the main constituents of blood :

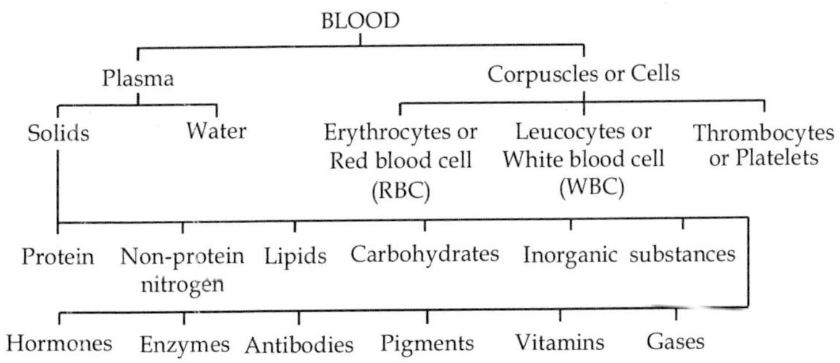

Functions of Blood

In the metazoan, the blood performs the functions of surrounding environment for the exchange and transportation performed by body fluid or cytoplasma in protozoa. Claude Bernard has defined blood as milieu interior or internal environment for the performance of cell functions. The common functions of blood are listed as follows:

1. Transportation of oxygen from lungs to cells in all parts of the body for cell respiration and metabolism.
2. Transportation of carbon dioxide from the cells to lungs for exhalation.
3. Transportation of metabolic waste products from the site of production to the organs of excretion like kidneys, lungs, skin and large intestine, etc.
4. Transportation of hormones from the organs of production to the target organs requiring the hormones for specific functions.
5. Transportation of enzymes.
6. Transportation of nutrients to tissues.
7. Maintenance of acid-base equilibrium of the body.
8. Maintenance of water balance of the tissue and also to provide protection from certain degree of dehydration.
9. Maintenance of a steady osmotic pressure in the tissues and body fluids (Homeostasis).
10. Thermoregulation of the body.
11. Haemostasis through coagulation mechanism.
12. Defence against microbial infections by phagocytosis.
13. To provide protection against dehydration by changing the shape of erythrocytes.

Physical Properties of Blood

Like other mammalian species the fresh blood of camelids is red, opaque and slightly alkaline fluid. It is slightly viscous and sticky and has characteristic odour of species. The taste of blood is salty. Main characteristics of the blood are listed as follows:

1. The colour of blood is variable due to the concentration of erythrocytes and haemoglobin. The arterial blood is bright red

due to the formation of oxyhaemoglobin, whereas venous blood is dark red due to reduced haemoglobin (Carbon dioxide containing blood).

2. There is characteristic odour in the blood due to the presence of volatile fatty acids.

3. The taste is somewhat salty due to the presence of inorganic salts of sodium and potassium.

4. The buffering capacity of blood is very high.

5. The temperature of fresh peripheral blood is almost similar to the body temperature, but slightly higher for the blood from deep seated vessels.

6. The osmolality of camel's blood increases with dehydration and drops after rehydration (Yagil *et al.,*, 1974). The blood has unusual high osmotic stability (Livne and Kuiper, 1973).

7. The specific gravity of camel blood is somewhat higher than many of the farm animals, although the erythrocytes are small. The specific gravity of dromedary's blood is 1.058 ± 0.009 to 1.054 ± 0.495 (Soliman and Slaker, 1967, Barakat and Abdel-Fattah, 1970). An increase in specific gravity occurs due to dehydration and it further increases immediately after rehydration but subsequently decreases to almost normal level after about 4 hours of rehydration (Yagil *et al.*, 1974).

8. The reaction of blood is slightly alkaline. An average 7.60 ± 0.03 pH reported by Soliman and Slaker (1967) is a little higher than pH 7.45 ± 0.008 (range, 7.1-7.6) observed by Barakat and Abdel-Fattah (1970). Still lower average values have been reported, i.e. pH 7.335± 0.026 and 7.341 ± 0.032 for the camel blood (Snow *et al.*, 1988). The values decreases to pH 6.984 ± 0.071 and 7.079 ± 0.05 after 4 and 5 km exercise at 20! atmospheric temperature.

9. Average clotting time of blood of the dromedary is 6.2 ± 0.02 minutes (Soliman and Slaker, 1967). Higher duration of 9-10 minutes for the dromedary and guanaco and 14.5 minutes for 11ama has been reported by Lewis (1976) but these values may not be considered normal because these were recorded on one or two individuals available in a zoo.

Homeostasis

The mechanism of blood for the maintenance of uniformity and stability in the extracellular fluid is known as homeostasis. The homeostasis is essential for the optimum function of cells and it is maintained by the interaction of several physiological functions like diffusion, active transport, concentration gredients, pressure gredients and regulatory mechanism of the nervous and endocrine systems. In the camel, there is very efficient water regulating mechanism involving mobilization of water from one compartment to another. The camel thus maintains its blood volume at the expense of body water during dehydration (Ghosal *et al.,* 1974).

Haemostasis

The control of bleeding is known as haemostasis. It may be natural or mechanical. The natural haemostais is effective in arresting the bleeding from the small vessels. This is caused by the formation of a haemostatic plug, which is formed by the aggregation of platelets followed by the deposition of fibrin. The erythrocytes and leucocytes are also present in the fibrin meshwork.

The bleeding from a vessel may cease when the internal and external hydrostatic pressure becomes equal. This can be produced by an increase in the external pressure either by accumulation of blood in the surrounding tissues or due to fall in intravascular pressure caysed by local vasoconstriction or by an effective fall in general blood pressure. The bleeding may be also arrested by the formation of a solid plug in the injured vessel due to the adhesion of the internal surfaces in small vessels. This mechanism is not effective in cases of haemophilia (encountered in some human families) where fibrin formation is deficient. Probably occurrence of such condition in the camelids is not yet known.

Blood Volume

The blood and plasma volume of dromedary camels of hot tropical deserts of India has been found to be higher in summer (dry hot) than in the winter (dry cold) season. The mean blood volume is 7.8 ± 0.16 per cent of the body weight in summer and 6.4 ± 0.70 per cent in winter. The mean plasma volume during the corresponding seasons is about 4.7 ± 0.14 and 3.8 ± 0.07 per cent of the body weight. In the camels, there is very efficient water regulation mechanism involving mobilization of water from one compartment to another. The camel, thus maintains its blood volume at the expense of body water during the dry season. In summer, intracellular fluid space is reduced to 8.85± 0.52 per cent of the body weight as compared to 9.98 ± 0.42 per cent in the winter (Ghosal *et al.,* 1974).

Blood Plasma

The colloidal fluid part from the uncoagulated blood after the sedimentation of blood cells in the anti-coagulent mixed blood is known as plasma.

Blood Serum

The fluid part of the blood separated after the coagulation of blood cells is known as serum. After clotting of the blood cells there is retraction of the clot causing liberation of the serum. It is similar to the plasma but does not contain fibrinogen, prothrombin and other factors associated with the formation of blood clot.

Blood Cells

Similar to the other mammalian species the camel's blood also contains three types of cells. These are erythrocytes or red blood corpuscles, leucocytes or white blood corpuscles and thrombocytes or platelets. The leucocytes are largest and the thrombocytes are smallest of the blood cells. Different types of blood cells are responsible for separate functions. The main function of RBC is gaseous exchange at the cellular level. The leucocytes are responsible for protective phagocytosis for controlling the population of harmful infectious micro-organisms and the platelets play important role in blood clotting.

Erythrocyte or Red Blood Cells (RBC)

The RBC of adult camel is elliptical and non-nucleated, and can drastically change in shape when running through the fine capillaries (Ponder *et al.,* 1928, Connelius *et al.,* 1962, Kohli, 1963). The RBC appears wafer like being thin and flat and exhibited slight and socytosis when viewed with the scanning electron microscope (Jain and Keelon, 1974). There is no apparent change in the shape of RBC due to dehydration but after rapid rehydration most of the erythrocytes become round (Yagil *et al.,* 1974).

The membrane of RBC possesses unusual high stability. The protection against the osmotic haemolysis afforded by added lipid to camel RBC is much less than that in the other mammals. The shift in osmotic fragility is also much less in the other mammals. The shift in osmotic fragility is also much less in comparison to human RBC. The osmotic potential of camel's RBC 278 mos mole is almost similar to other species. Thus, the stability of the camel's RBC is related to the membrane properties causing unusual slow haemolysis. The RBCs of camel are at least three times more resistant than the RBC of human, sheep and rat against the ultrasonic haemolysis (Livne and Kuiper, 1973). This is probably due to the abundance of protein in the RBC membrane, which is particularly rich in integral proteins and in intramembranous particles. It appears to be a dominant structural feature stabilizing the erythrocyte membrane in the camels (Eitan *et al.,* 1976). The fragility and osmolality of the RBC increases with the dehydration and decreases after rehydration (Yagil *et al.,* 1974). The RBC of camels have lower water content and a much higher oxygen affinity and a lower electrolyte (Na and K) levels than the RBC of other farm animals (Little *et al.,* 1970).

Dimensions of Erythrocytes

The dimension of camelid's erythrocytes has been reported to be quite variable. The average dimension of RBC is 7.5 × 4.0μm (Cornelius and Kaneko, 1968). The long axis is 6.5 to 11.25 μm and short axis is 3.75 to 6.25 μm with an average dimension of 7.60 × 4.47 μm. The common size of RBC is 7.3 to 7.69 μm long and 4.3 to 4.59 μm wide in the Indian and Arabian camels (Kohli, 1963, Yagil *et al.,* 1974). The average size of the RBC of 11amoids (Lama Glama and L. guanaco) is somewhat larger (9 × 4) than the dromedaries, 7.5 × 4.0 μm (Lewis, 1976). However, these observations are limited to only one or two individuals of each species kept in a zoo. The average thickness of RBC of dromedary has been reported to be 2.5 μm (Abdel-Gadir *et al.,* 1979). The average area of the normal RBC of dromedary is 50.6 um^2. The dimension as well as area of RBC are significantly reduced to 8.8 ± 0.2× 5.4± 0.1 μm and 37.3 ± 1.1 μm^2 without any significant change in the shape even after 7 days of dehydration. Rehydration does not cause significant change in the shape and size upto 30 minutes but after about 4 hours of rehydration, the shape of RBC becomes round due to significant reduction in long axis to 7.9 ± 0.2 μm and increase in short axis to 6.7 ± 0.2 μm. The average area is 38.9 ± 1.3 μm^2 after 30 minutes and 40.8 ± 1.3 μm^2 after 4 hours of rehydration (Yagil *et al.,* 1974).

Erythrocyte Count

A large variation in the RBC count has been observed in the blood of different species of camelidae. Besides age and sex, the variation is more influenced by the agro-climatic conditions including availability of drinking water and quality as well as quantity of the feeds and fodder supply. Inadequate availability of feeds causes unthriftiness, whereas scarcity of drinking water leads to dehydration of various degree causing haemoconcentration. The RBC count in dromedary ranges from 4.2 to 12.5 million per cubic millimeter (Soni and Aggarwala, 1958, Soliman and Slaker, 1967, Barakat and Abdel-Fattah, 1970, Sharma *et al.*, 1973, Yagil *et al.*, 1974, Lewis, 1976, Ghodsian *et al.*, 1978, Musa and Mukhtar, 1982). The number of RBC has been found to be somewhat higher in females (8.25-9.75, mean 8.91 million per mm^3) than in the male dromedaries (6.75-10.32, mean 8.48 million per mm^3) as observed by Adam *et al.*, (1974). But, another observation shows higher RBC count (10.22 million per mm^3) in the adult dromedary of 5-9 years of age than the 8.67 million in the young females of 1.5-4 years of age (Ateeq *et al.*, 1984). No change in RBC count has been observed upto 7 days dehydration but the number of cells decreased sharply following the drinking of large volume of water after dehydration (Yagil *et al.*, 1974). This is probably due to haemodilution (Etzion *et al.*, 1984). In the bactrian or double-humped camels, the RBC count in a single female has been observed to be 11.02 million per mm^3 (bartels *et al.*, 1963). It is more or less similar to dromedary in llama but little higher in guanaco (Lewis, 1976). The RBC count in the juveniles of the cameloids is higher than the adults (Hawkey and Gulland, 1982). Physical exercise in the racing camels has no significant effect on RBC count (Snow *et al.*, 1988).

Erythrocyte Sedimentation Rate (ESR)

The rate of setting of the RBC measured with the help of a Westergren sedimentation tube per unit of time is known as ESR which indicates the suspension stability of the erythrocytes. For this purpose anticoagulent added blood is used, and ESR is measured as mm per hour. The setting of RBCs is resisted by the surface area of the falling particles and ESR depends on the rate of ouleaus (like pile of same coins) formation of the RBCs. Zero ESR has been observed for the first hour in dromedary, llama and guanaco (Sharma *et al.*, 1973, Hawkey and Gulland, 1988). However, in the female dromedary exclusively the ESR was 1.0 + 0.62 mm during the first hour and 2.5 mm during the second hour (Soliman and Slaker, 1967). After 6 hours, the ESR in adult Indian camels has been found to be 6.3 + 0.97 mm (Sharma *et al.*, 1973). This was closer to values ranging from 5 to10 mm (mean 7mm) after 6 hours (Bhatt and Kohli, 1959). The average ESR has been reported to be 0.9 (0.5-2.0), 2.0 (1-4), 3.4 (2-6), 4.6 (3-8), 5.7 (3.5-9.0), 7.0 (5-10) and 8.1 (6.5-10.5) mm afer 1, 2, 3, 4, 5, 6 and 7 hours of gravitational sedimentation respectively in the Bikaneri camels (Bhatt and Kohli, 1959). A slight increase in ESR has been observed in racing camels after 4 and 5 km race at 20°C atmospheric temperature. The values before the race were 0.326 and 0.338 mm during one hour for the camels used for 4 and 5 km race respectively, which rose to 0.34 and 0.35 mm in one hour after race in the corresponding camels (Snow *et al.*, 1983).

A decrease in ESR due to dehydration and an increased after rehydration has been observed in the dromedaries. The ESR is the characteristic of the blood cells of a species and it does not change significantly when the cells are suspended in the plasma of other species like man and chicken (Etzion *et al.*, 1985).

Haematocrit or Packed Cell Volume (PCV)

A large variation in haematocrit values may be due to various degree of dehydration in the camels and also due to the differences in the environment and breeds (Table 2).

Table 2. Haematocrit (%) values in different species of the camelids at different age and in two sexes.

Species	Age	Sex	PCV (%)	Sources
Drome dary	Adult	Female	43.0 + 1.10	Soliman & Slaker (1967)
	Adult		36.9 + 4.14	Sharma *et al.*, (1973)
	Adult, normal		28.5	Yagil *et al.*, (1974)
	dehydrated		26.0	
	rehydrated (4 h)		23.0	
	Adult	Male	35.4 (28-41)	Adam *et al.*, (1974)
		Female	34.7 (27-42)	
	Adult		27.9 + 1.54	Agar *et al.*, (1982)
	Adult		34.8	Repoport & Quest (1941)
Bactrian	Adult	Female	35.2	Bartels *et al.*, (1963)

Drome dary	Adult	23.7-37.0	Lewis (1976)
Llama	Adult	22.3	
Guanaco	Adult	31.7	
Llama	Adult	30.0 (27-36)	Hawkey & Gulland (1988)
	Juvenile	31.0 (27-35)	
Guanaco	Adult	36.0 (28-42)	
	Juvenile	36.0 (34-37)	

The variation in PCV values observed between the different studies clearly shows the need of more extensive studies for establishing the normal values considering various factors like age, sex, species and environment, etc.

Life Span of Erythrocyte

The average time of survival of the RBC of dromedary is about 90 days in winter and 120 days in summer season. In the cases of chronic dehydration, a significant increase in the survival of RBCs upto 150 days has been observed (Yagil *et al.*, 1974). The average life span of the RBC of guanaco ranges from 225 to 235 days and occassionally it may be over 240 days (Cornelius and Kaneko, 1962).

Critical Haemolytic Volume of the RBC

The values of critical haemolytic volume of RBC of one-humped camel is 2 X Vo (Perk *et al.*, 1963) against 1.8 X Vo for the humans (Seeman *et al.*, 1969). As high as 240 per cent rise in the volume of the erythrocytes of the camels may occur without rupture (Perk, 1963). This property of camel's RBC helps in the accumulation of the large volume of water during sudden rehydration.

Fate of the Erythrocytes

The erythrocytes are regularly destroyed by the reticulo-endothelial system after maturity. the haemoglobin, thus released is disintegrated into globin, ferrous ion (Fe^{++}) and porphyrin. The iron released is trapped by apoferritin to form ferritin, which is subsequently utilized for the formation of fresh haemoglobin.

The porphyrin released from the break down of RBCs is converted into biliverdin by the reticulo-endothelial system, which may be reduced to bilirubin. Both are the bile pigments. These pigments enter into the intestine in bile pigments. These pigments enter into the intestine in bile where they are further reduced by the intestinal microflora into stercobilinogen, which may be oxidised to stercobolin. The latter two are faecal pigments. A part of stercobilinogen may be again absorbed and carried to the liver by the ported circulation. In liver, a portion of stercobilinogen is reconverted into the bile pigment and remaining is excreted in the urine as almost colourless urobilinogen. On exposure to air the urinary urobilinogen turns yellow due to its oxidation in yellow urobilin.

The Membrane of Red Blood Cell

The membrane of RBC is formed of mainly proteins and lipids in the ratio of 3.4 : 1 in the dromedaries. The membrane proteins are of two types, i.e. integral proteins and peripheral proteins. The RBC's membrane is particularly rich in integral proteins and in intramembranous particles. This dominant structural characteristic is responsible for estabilishing the RBC membrane. The peripheral protein is about 12 per cent and the integral protein is about 88 per cent of the cell membrane proteins (Eitan *et al.*, 1976, Aloni *et al.*, 1977).

The unusual high osmotic stability of the camel's RBC membrane is due to the compositional difference from the other species. The RBC of camel is at least 3 times more resistant than the RBC of human, sheep and rat against the ultrasonic haemolysis. The total lipids in RBC of camel is 6.05 + 0.60 mg per ml PCV and the ratio of phospholipids and cholesterol is almost equal. Perhaps only information available on amino acids composition of the RBC membrane (Table 3) shows difference in the percentage of concentration of some of the amino acids from the RBC membrane of human (Livne and Kuiper, 1973).

Table 3. Percentage composition of amino acids in the RBC membrane of camel and human cells.

Amino acids	Camels RBC	Human's RBC
Alanine	7.7	8.4
Arginine	6.0	5.0
Aapartic acid	7.9	8.1
Cystine (half)	0.7	0.7
Glutamic acid	12.3	13.0

Histidine	2.7	2.9
Isoleucine	4.4	4.3
Leucine	12.2	11.8
Lysine	5.7	5.5
Methionine	2.0	2.6
Phenylalanine	4.5	5.0
Proline	6.8	5.3
Threonine	4.9	5.4
Tryptophane	+	+
Tyrosine	2.6	2.7
Valine	6.8	6.8

Haemoglobin

A great variation has been found in the values of haemoglobin (Hb) of the camelids, which may be due to several factors like nutritional variations, dehydration, breeds, species, sex, age and climatic conditions besides the non-pathological conditions. The Hb values of the dromedaries ranges from 8.99 to 19.01 g per cent. Average values reproted by different workers in dromedaries are 13.20 + 0.81 (Soliman and Slakrt, 1967), 13.05 + 0.12 (Barakat and Abdel-Fattah, 1970), 9.88 + 0.8 (Sharma *et al.*, 1973), 12.5 + 0.82 (Agar and Suzuki, 1982), 11.6 + 2.5 (Missa and Mukhtar, 1982) and 14.5 + 1.50 (Al-Ali *et al.*, 1988). The average Hb in female camels 14.23 (range, 9.3 to 19.01) g per cent is slightly higher than 13.95 (range, 11.09 to 18.73) g per cent in the male dromedaries (Adam *et al.*, 1974). A marginal increase in Hb content from 15.1 + 1.1 g before exercise to 15.4 + 1.2 g per cent after 4 km racing, and from 15.7 + 0.7 g before exercise to 16.1 + 0.3 g per cent after 5 km racing has been observed by Snow *et al.*, (1988). This may be due to haemoconcentration caused by some dehydration during the exercise. Dehydration has apparent effect on the Hb content, which reduced from 15.5 g per cent in normally watered camels to 12.1 g per cent after 7 days of dehydration and further fell to 6.9 g per cent after 4 hours of rehydration (Yagil *et al.*, 1974). There is adjustment difference between the former and the latter conditions. A decline in Hb conent of the male camel's blood occours during the breeding season, which is winter in India. This phenomenon is not associated with either the oxygen consumption or the scarcity of drinking water (Khan and Kohli, 1978).

The haemoglobin value of one female llama of about 1.5 year of age has been observed to be 18.8 g per cent and in one bactrian camel of about 300 kg body weight it was 15.8 g per cent (Bartels *et al.*, 1963). The average of 14 adult and 10 juvenile llamas was 13.7 + 2.4 g and 13.5 + 0.9 g per cent respectively. A higher value of 15.7 + 1.7 g in the adult guanacos and 15.9 + 0.7 g in juvenile guanacos has vbeen recorded (Hawkeyd and Gulland, 1988).

About 95-99 per cent native Hb of camel blood is alkali resistant and soluble in 2.94 molar solution of K_2HP0_4 or K_2HP0_4 buffer. The spontaneous formation of methaemoglobin in camel's blood is very slow (Lin *et al.*, 1976). In the dromedary, glycosylated Hb is about 5.5 + 0.38 per cent and ranges from 5 to 6.35 per cent (Alayash and Wilson, 1988). The concentration of Hb in RBC of camel is higher than the many farm animals. This compensate the reduction in pulmonary gaseous exchange (Siebert and Macfarlane, 1975). The Hb of camel possesses a great affinity for the oxygen. This results in higher oxygen uptake per unit volume of RBCs and this property is more advantageous for the smaller camelids like llama, alpaca, guanaco and vicuna living under the low oxygen pressure at high altitudes (Bartels *et al.*, 1963).

Mean Corpuscular Volume (MCV)

An earlier value of MCV, 59.99 + 1.40 μm^3 in the adult dromedary female (Soliman and Slaker, 1967) is much higher than 31.05 + 6.42 μm^3 (Sharma *et al.*, 1973) and 43.6 + 8.9 μm^3 (Musa and Mukhtar, 1982) observed in subsequent studies. Still lower value of 28.5 μm^3 has been observed by Yagil *et al.*, (1974), which further declined to 26 μm^3 after 7 days of dehydration but returned to somewhat higher level, i.e. 33.3 μm^3 after 4 hours of sudden rehydration. The values for the male and female Sudanese dromedaries are 42.0 (34.7 to 46.6) and 38.9 (30 to 45.2) μm^3 respectively (Adam *et al.*, 1974). In the new world cameloids, the values of MCV is lower than the dromedary. In the adult and juvenile llamas, it is 26.9 + 1.3 and 25.8 + 1.8 μm^3; and in the adult and juvenile guanacos 27.5 + 1.7 and 25.6 + 1.7 μm^3 respectively (Hawkey and Gulland, 1988).

Mean Corpuscular Haemoglobin (MCH)

The value of MCH ranges from 8.95 + 1.79 to 18.32 + 0.89 pg in the dromedaries of different countries (Soliman and Slaker, 1967, Sharma *et al.*, 1973, Yagil *et al.*, 1974). Lewis (1976) reported 22, 22 and 28 pg MCH in dromedary, guanaco and llama respectively.

however, average values of 14 adult and 10 juvenile llamas were 12.0 + 0.6 and 11.4 + 0.5 pg; and those of 17 adult and 5 juvenile guanacos were 12.1 + 0.8 and 11.2 + 0.7 pg, respectively (Hawkey and Gulland, 1988).

Mean Corpuscular Haemoglobin Concentration (MCHC)

Like other haematological value, there is also large variation in the values of MCHC. Different workers have reported different values, viz., 30.7 + 1.11 g per cent (Sharma *et al.*, 1973), 54.4 g per cent (Yagil *et al.*, 1974) and 43.9 + 6.6 g per cent (Musa and Mukhtar, 1982). A slight fall from 54.4 g per cent normal to 46.5 g per cent after 7 days of dehydration and a further fall to 44.4 g per cent after 4 hours of rehydration in MCHC has been observed (Yagil *et al.*, 1974). In the male dromedary 42.9 (40.3 to 46.8) and in females 41.2 (35.0 to 48.9) g per cent has been observed by Adam *et al.*, (1974). In a single individual of dromedary, guanaco and llama, the value of MCHC has been reported to be 57, 51 and 73 g per cent (Lewis, 1976). The average MCHC in the adult and juvenile llamas were 44.8 + 2.3 and 44.5 + 2.4 g per cent; and the adult and juvenile guanacos 43.8 + 2.0 and 43.9 + 0.6 g per cent, respectively (Hawkey and Gulland, 1988).

Leucocytes or White Blood Corpuscles (WBC)

Like erythrocytes, a great variation has been also observed in the leucocytes count in camel blood. It ranges from 11.0 to 19.2 thousand per μl of blood. The average WBC count in dromedary reported by different workers are 12.5 + 0.82 (Soliman and Slaker, 1967), 15.04 + 0.34 (Barakat and Abdel-Fattah, 1970), 15.16 + 0.68 (Sharma *et al.*, 1973), 13.23 (Abdel-Gadir *et al.*, 1979) and 12.6 + 5.2 (Musa and Mukhtar, 1982). About 2.7 to 7.5 per cent higher WBC count has been observed in the female than the male dromedary (Adam *et al.*, 1974, Ateeq *et al.*, 1984). A marginal increase of 2 and 6.8 per cent has been also observed in the racing camels after 4 and 5 km exercise respectively (Snow *et al.*, 1988). The WBC count in a guanaco and a llama was 17.5 and 13.9 thousand per microlitre of blood respectively (Lewis, 1976). However, in another observations on more number of animals, the WBC count has been found to be much lower than the dromedary. The values are 8.7 + 1.4, 12.4 + 3.7, 10.4 + 3.2 and 13.3 + 3.4 thousands per microlitre of blood in the adult llama, juvenile llama, adult guanaco and juvenile guanaco respectively (Howkey and Gulland, 1988). No apparent role of WBC has been so far observed in the adaptation of the camelids in the harsh environemnt of the arid and semi-arid regions.

Contradictory findings are available about the ratio of the lymphocytes and neutrophils in the population of WBC of dromedary. A higher proportion of lymphocytes ranging from 50 to 78 per cent (mean, 66.57 + 0.82) has been reported by Barakat and Abdel-Fattah (1970) and 63.0 + 2.12 per cent by Soliman and Slaker (1967). On the other hand, lower values of 39.6 + 2.92 and 33.9 + 11.4 per cent have been reported by Sharma *et al.*, (1973) and Musa and Mukhtar (1982). The lymphocytes are little less and eosinophils are little more in the female than the male dromedaries (Adam *et al.*, 1974). Some values of leucocytes are given in table 4). In the llamas and guanacos also, the ratio of neutrophils was higher than the lymphocytes in adults but more or less similar in the juveniles (Hawkey and Gulland, 1988).

Size of the White Blood Cells

The average length of the WBC of Indian desert camel is 7.485 + 0.0272 μm and width is 4.433 + 0.0177 μm. The average long axis of the neutrophils, eosinophils, lymphocytes and monocytes is 13.172 + 0.0953, 15.266 + 0.0911, 11.930 + 0.1824 and 15.891 + 0.4451 μm respectively (Kohli, 1963).

Characteristics of the Leucocytes

1. The WBCs are somewhat larger in size than the RBCs.
2. The WBCs are nucleated.
3. Population of WBC in the circulation is much less than the RBC.
4. Leucocytes do not contain haemoglobin.
5. Leucocytes are active like amoeba and have phagocytic character which helps in controlling infectious diseases.
6. WBCs are of different types, which are classified as (i) granulocytes consisting of neutrophils, eosinophils and basophils, and (ii) agranulocytes consisting of lymphocytes and monocytes.
7. The origin of WBC is extravascular.
8. They consume oxygen and glucose and produce lactic acid.
9. Life span of WBC is usually shorter than the RBC, but for the camelidae probably it is not known.

Table 4. Mean values of leucocytes in the blood of the camelids.

Leucocytes	Dromedary camels						Llamas 5		Guanacos 5	
	1	2	3	4	Male	Female	Adult	Juvenile	Adult	Juvenile
Leucocyte (X 10^3)	12.50 + 0.82	15.04 + 0.34	15.16 + 0.68	12.60 + 5.20		+ 0.4	8.7 + 3.7	12.4 + 3.2	10.4 + 3.4	13.3
Lymphocyte, %	63.0 + 2.12	66.6 + 0.82	39.6 + 8.92	33.9 + 11.4	45.4	45.8	27.4	51.2	30.0	46.5
Neutrophil, %	31.7 + 1.12	26.2 + 0.75	43.8 + 7.26	55.1 + 5.2	44.6	42.6	61.9	41.1	62.0	47.2
Eosinophil, %	2.2 + 0.04	3.4 + 0.23	13.8 + 6.64	1.5 + 0.8	4.6	7.2	3.6	1.5	1.0	1
Monocytes, %	2.4 + 0.32	2.8 + 0.13	2.6 + 0.23	4.5 + 1.6	5.2	4.0	7.1	4.7	7.0	5.6
Basophils, %	0.7 + 0.01	1	0.2 + 0.14	0.16 + 0.50	0.0	0.4	1	1.5	1	0.0

Sources: 1- Soliman & Slaker, 1967; 2- Barakat & Abdel-Fattah, 1970; 3- Sharma *et al.*, 1973; 4- Musa & Mukhtar, 1982; and 5- Hawkey & Gulland, 1988.

Functions of the Leucocytes

Different kinds of leucocytes play different role in the body. However, main functions of WBC is to provide defence against the invaders for the protection of normal health. The various functions performed by different WBC cells are listed as follows:

1. Polymorphs and monocytes are highly phagocytic and can pass out of the blood vessels into the surrounding tissues by diapedesis, the process of amoeboid movement of polymorphs and monosites at the side of inflammation caused by bactria. The leucotoxins, liberated due to pathological reaction of invader bacteria with the tissue cells, attract WBC to the site of bacterial infection. The phagocytic characteristic of the leucocytes is due to the presence of opsonin in the blood serum. Washed WBCs do not engulf bacteria but phagocytosis is again started on adding serum in the washed WBC and bacteria mixture.
2. Leucocytes destroy dead cells debris by ingestion and subsequent liquification.
3. Lymphocytes and monocytes also produce certain growth producing substances like trephones from the plasma protein.
4. Due to disintegration of the lymphocytes, the protein liberated is added to the plasma protein in the circulation.
5. Lymphocytes synthesise antibodies of game-globin type, which protects tissue cells from the bacterial toxins and make bacteria as far as possible harmless. These antibodies are bacteriolysins, anti-toxins and agglutinins. Higher population of infective bacteria in the body stimulate higher production of lymphocytes.
6. Basophils participate in the manufacture of heparin.

Fate of the Leucocytes

All the white blood cells remain in circulation for a short life after their formation and then they are disintegrated in the blood strosm. The WBC involved in bactericidal activities are also disintegrated and then ingested by the reticulo-endothelial cells.

Thrombocytes / Platelets

The thrombocytes of the camelids are smaller and more flat than the platelets of many other mammalians. The diameter of the platelets of dromedary is 1-2 μm and that of llama is 2 μm. The platelets count in a dromedary and a llama has been reported to be 1730 X 10^3 and 370 X 10^3 per microlitre respectively (Lewis, 1976). However, these values need further confirmation through the observations on larger population. Average platelets count per ml of blood in the adult and juveniles of llamas and guanacos has been observed to be 332 ± 7 and 500 ± 229, and 282 ± 108 and 419 ± 43 million, respectively (Hawkey and Gulland, 1988). The latter values show a great variation in the population. However, mean counts were higher for the juveniles in both the species.

Functions of the Throbocytes

1. At the time of blood shading due to trauma or any other reason, the platelets disintegrate and liberate platelet factor, lipoid thromboplastin, which initiates the clotting of blood. A plasma factor, thrombocytolysin has been found to be responsible for the lysis of the platelets during bleeding.
2. The platelets adhere to the injured endothelial surface of the capillaries and help the repair of the endothelium of the capillary. Platelets cluming also helps in repair.
3. The thrombocytes help in retraction of the blood clot, which becomes tougher, non-solid and elastic.

Blood Plasma

The fluid portion of uncoagulated blood containing soluble and colloidal particles is known as plasma. It may be colourless to yellowish depending on its volume, bilirubin content and amount of dietary pigments like carotenes.

Blood Serum

The fluid sparated from the coagulation of blood after the retraction of blood clot is known as serum. It is similar to plasma from which fibrinogen and other clotting factors have been removed into the blood clot during the process of coagulation of the blood.

Composition of Blood Plasma

About 60-70 per cent of blood is plasma, and the plasma contains about 90 per cent water and 10 per cent solids. The solid portion of the plasma is formed of proteins, lipids, sugars, inorganic substances, hormones, enzymes, antibodies, pigments and gases.

Nitrogenous Fractions of the Blood

Like other mammalian species, the various nitrogenous fractions of the camel's blood are protein, urea, uric acid, ammonia, creatine, creatinine and amino acids. Traces of xanthine and hypoxanthine may be also present. The values of nitrogenous fractions are mostly reported in the serum of blood which excludes fibrinogen and prothrombin. A large variation from 4.8 to more than 7.9 g protein per 100 ml of serum has been observed in the dromedaries of different countries (Soliman and Slaker, 1967, Baraat and Abdel-Fattah, 1970, Lewis, 1976). Influence of reproductive stages in the females (Ateeq *et al.*, 1984, Kouider *et al.*, 1988), sex (Lassen *et al.*, 1986) and age (Abdo *et al.*, 1987) has been observed in the serum protein content (Table 5). The fibrinogen content in the Indian dromedary is about 255 ± 7.9 (range, 241-284) mg per 100 ml of blood (Kumar *et al.*, 1961). The concentration of fibrinogen in the adults and juveniles of the llama and guanaco is 1.9 ± 0.5 and 2.3 ± 0.4 and 2.9 ± 0.8 and 2.5 ± 0.4 g per litre of blood respectively (Hawkey and Gulland, 1988).

Table 5. Serum protein content in the blood of camelids.

Type of camelid	Serum protein (mg/dl)	Source
Dromedary		
Indian camel	6.4 ± 0.55 (5.6-7.85)	Kumar *et al.*, 1961
do, Summer	6.3 ± 0.15	Ghosal *et al.*, 1974
do, Winter	6.8 ± 0.12	
Arabian camel,		Abdo *et al.*, 1987
below 3 years age	6.10 ± 0.24	
below 5 years age	5.82 ± 0.32	
Normal herd	6.42 ± 0.004 (5.47-7.30)	Barakat & Abdel-Fattah, 1970
Adult female	7.02 ± 0.19	Soliman & Slaker, 1967
Quiseent female	6.53 ± 0.44	Kouider *et al.*, 1988
Breeding female	7.84 ± 0.61	-do-
Non-pregnant female	6.1	Ateeq *et al.*, 1984
Pregnant female	7.1	-do-
Non-pregnant female	13.39 (in blood)	Elthony *et al.*, 1986
Pregnant female	16.64 do	-do-
Racing camels	–	Snow *et al.*, 1988

before excercise	6.54 ± 0.24	
after 4 km race	6.78 ± 0.26	
after 5 km race	6.90 ± 0.30	
before exercise	6.80 ± 0.30	
Bactrian camel	8.5	Kchouk & Durand, 1958
New World Cameloids		
Llama	6.0	Lewis, 1986
Guanaco	5.4	-do-
Llama flock	5.9 ± 0.4	Lassen *et al.*, 1986
Llama, males	5.8 ± 0.5 (5.0 - 7.8)	-do-
Llama, females	6.0 ± 0.4 (5.3 - 6.9)	-do-

Serum Protein Fractions

The serum protein is formed of albumin and globulins. The proportion of albumin is normally higher than the globulins irrespective of species, age, sex and dehydration condition of the camelids (Lewis, 1976, Mohamed *et al.*, 1983, Lassen *et al.*, 1986, Abdo *et al.*, 1987). However, a study on the bacterian camels (Kchouk and Durand, 1958) and another on the Indian dromedaries (Kumar *et al.*, 1961) has shown a reverse trend. This needs further conformation and also investigations about the factors responsible for the reversal, if any, of the normal pattern of the serum protein fractions. In the male dromedary, albumin content is higher and albumin : globulins ration is lower than the females. However, total blood proteins and globulins are non-significantly affected by the sex (Chiericato *et al.*, 1986). A marginal increase in the serum albumin content has been observed after exercise in the racing dromedaries (Snow *et al.*, 1988). The foetal serum protein increases with the foetal development and foetal serum albumin increases more rapidly in the late pregnancy. Initially at about 1-20 cm crown-rump (CR) length of foetii, the content of serum alpha-globulin is more than half of the total serum protein, thereafter it decreases gradually. Foetal beta-globulin has been found to be maximum at about 21-60 cm CR length, which decreases afterwards. Foetal gama-globulin increases gradually with advancing pregnancy and the newborns are not totally agamaglobulinaemic. The maternal serum protein and its fractions were almost constant during the pregancy (Salib and Saleh, 1984). The information on serum protein fractions are summarised in Table 6.

Table 6. Per cent serum protein fractions and albumin: globulins (A:G) ratio in camelids.

S.No.	Species	Albumin	Alpha 1-globulin	Alpha 2-globulin	Beta-globulin	Gamma globulin	A:G ratio	Source
1.	Bacterian	41.5 ± 4	4.8 ± 1.2	9.3 ± 2.0	17.2 ± 1.5	27.3 ± 3.0	42:58	Kchouk & Durrand, 1958
2.	Dromedary	35.8 ± 0.83 (31.5-39.4)	5.3 ± 0.23 (3.8-6.3)	19.1 ± 2.3 (14.6-24.2)	30.9 ± 0.18 (26.9-34.7)	7.4 ± 1.43 (6.4-12.8)	36:64	Kumar *et al.*, 1961
3.	do, below 3 yr	59.0	2.0		18.33	20.67	59:41	Abdo *et al.*, 1987
	above 3 yr	62.0	2.0		15.40	20.00	62:38	-do-
4.	Dromedary	70.8	4.2	8.3	12.50	4.20	71:29	Lewis, 1976
	Guanaco	57.4	9.3	13.0	13.00	7.40	57:43	-do-
	Llama	57.5	2.2	9.7	22.80	7.50	58:42	-do-
5.	Llama	59.0	-	-	-	-	59:41	Lassen *et al.*, 1986
	do, male	58.6	-	-	-	-	59:41	-do-
	do, female	60.0	-	-	-	-	60:40	-do-

Other Nitrogenous Constituents of Blood

The non-protein nitrogenous constituents of the blood are urea, ammonia, uric acid, creatine, creatinine and amino acids. The values observed by various workers in different camelids are summarised in Table 7. About 4-6 per cent increase in blood urea, 315-445 per cent increase in blood ammonia and 123-130 per cent increase in blood creatinine has been observed in the racing camels after 4-5 km exercise at 20°C atmospheric temperature (Snow *et al.*, 1988).

Plasma Lipids

Total lipids in the blood plasma of the dromedary are 104.4 ± 14.8 mg per 100 ml (Al-ali *et al.*, 1988). It has been found to be a little higher (3.02 ± 0.23 g/l) during the quiscent period than the 2.77 ± 0.16 g per litre during the breeding season (Kouider *et al.*, 1988). The values of phospholipids, alpha-lipoprotein, beta-lipoprotein and '0' fraction of the lipoprotein are 329 ± 11.30 (300-388), 22.4 ± 1.50 (17-32), 32.5 ± 1.36 (27-39) and 44.9 ± 2.17 (39-54) mg per 100 ml of serum respectively in the Indian camels (Kumar *et al.*, 1961). A significant increase in the concentration of lactic acid and triglycerides, and decrease in free-fatty acids (Table 8) in the racing camels has been observed after exercise (Snow *et al.*, 1988).

The concentration of total and free cholesterol has been observed to be 181 ± 3.9 (167-195) mg and 62 ± 1.90 (52-72) mg per 100 ml of serum in the Indian camels (Kumar, 1961). A wider range of 63.16 to total cholesterol content 30.5 ± mg per dl observed by is much lower than the earlier values but similar to the single observation of Lewis (1976), which 45 mg per dl for both dromedary and llama. The cholesterol content has been found to be higher (1.87 ± 0.19 m.ml/1) during the breeding season than the 1.49 ± 0.15 m.mole/1 in the quiscent period (Kouider, 1988). In the older female dromedaries of 5 to 9 years of age, a higher value of cholesterol, i.e. 55.7 mg/dl was observed. It was only 39.1 mg/dl in the younger females of 1.5 to 4 years of age (Ateeq *et al.*, 1984).

Table 7. Values of non-protein nitrogenous (NPN) constituents in the blood of camelids.

Species	Urea-N (mg/dl)	Uric acid-N (mg/dl)	Ctreatine (mg/dl)	Creatinine (mg/dl)	NPN (mg/dl)	Amino acid-N (mg/dl)	Source
Dromedary,							
female	9.2		2.82 ± 0.21	0.74 ± 0.03	-	-	Soliman & Slaker, 1967
Dromedary	9.7 ± 0.40	0.70 ± 0.05	2.90 ± 0.21	2.20 ± 0.31	30.00 ± 2.00	18.0 ± 1.50	Kumar *et al.*, 1961
do	12.0 ± 3.86	0.14 ± 0.004	0.62 ± 0.002	2.05 ± 0.10	26.04 ± 1.64	-	Barakat & Abdel-Fattah, 1970
do, male -							
young (1.5-4)	17.3						Ateeq *et al.*, 1984
adult (5-9 yr)	15.2						-do-
Dromedary	10.0	0.25		1.0			Lewis, 1976
Llama	23.0	1		1.7			do
Llama	27.0 ± 6.0			2.3			Lassen *et al.*, 1986
do, male	26.0 ± 6.0 (13-39)		2.4 ± 0.4				-do-
do, female	28.0 ± 6.0 (15-43)			2.2 ± 0.5			-do-

Table 8. Effect of exercise on some blood lipids.

Blood lipids	4 km racing		5 km racing	
(m.mol/l)	Before	After	Before	After
Triglycerides	0.28 ± 0.19	0.61 ± 0.22	0.26 ± 0.09	0.59 ± 0.15
Lactate	0.80 ± 0.50	24.3 ± 3.2	2.00 ± 0.60	21.4 ± 2.70
Free fatty acids	1.09 ± 0.32	0.23 ± 0.07	1.04 ± 0.41	0.21 ± 0.11

Blood Sugar

A great variation has been observed in the blood glucose content in the camelids. It is about 48 mg/ dl in whole blood and 108 mg/ dl in serum (Albritton, 1952). In the whole blood of Indian camels, glucose cotnent ranges frome 86.3 to 128.4 mg with an average of 110.1 ± 1.8 mg/ dl (Lal *et al.*, 1962). In serum it ranges from 80 to 140 mg/ dl. The other values of serum glucose content are 83 mg/ dl (Kchouk and Durand, 1958), 80 ± 2.22 mg/ dl (Soliman and Slaker, 1967), 104.13 ± 0.94 mg/ dl (Barakat and Abdel-Fattah, 1970) and 138 ± 17.7 mg/ dl (Al-Ali *et al.*, 1988). Single value 205 mg/ dl in dromedary was much higher and also higher than 106 mg/ dl blood glucose found in a single llama (Lewis, 1976). A significant fall in the serum glucose level due to rise in atomospheric temperature has been observed, which fell down to 99.2 ± 2.9 mg/ dl at 40°C from the initial 104.8 ± 8.1 mg/ dl at 25°C in the dromedaries (Kouider and Kolb, 1982). The effect of sex is not significant in the dromedaries (Chiericato *et al.*, 1986), but in the male llamas the level of blood glucose 136 ± 31 (97-223) ml/ dl has been found to be higher than 112 ± 17 (94-156) mg/dl in the female llamas (Lassen *et al.*, 1988).

A significant rise in blood glucose content due to race (exercise) has been observed in the dromedaries. The blood glucose level 6.8 ± 0.5 m.mol/1 before exercise in race camels rose to 11.7 ± 1.3 m.mol/1 after 4 km racing. In another group, it rose from 7.4 ± 0.4 m.mol/1 to 13.2 ± 2.5 m.mol/1 after 5 km racing at 20°C atmospheric temperature (Snow *et al.*, 1988).

Inorganic Constituents of Blood

Several inorganic compounds and ions are the normal constituents of the blood plasma and cells. So far, values of limited number of the inorganic constituents are known in the blood of the camelids. Phosphorus is found both in the organic as well as inorganic (Pi) form in the blood. In the blood of the bacterian camels, organic phosphorus is about 54.1 μg and Pi is 5.6 mg/ dl (Rapoport and Guest, 1941). In the blood of the Indian camels, Pi is about 7.18 ± 0.9

(5.45-8.20) mg/dl (Bhatt and Kohli, 1962) and in the Arabian camels it is about 8.4 ± 1.7 mg/dl (Al-Ali *et al.*, 1988).

The blood calcium level in the Egyptian dromedaries of various age and reporductive groups is about 10.65 ± 0.02 (9.5-11.3) mg/dl in young males; 11.10 (10.5-12.5) mg/dl in young females; 10.64 ± 0.02 (8.8-12.2) mg/dl in adult males; 10.72 ± 0.21 (9.3-12.2) mg/dl in non-pregnant adult females; and 10.37 ± 0.01 (9.4-11.7) mg/dl in pregnant females (Ayoub *et al.*, 1960). Another observations reported about 12.4 ± 0.09 (9.3-15.2) mg/dl calcium in the blood of normal camels (Barakat and Abdel-Fattah, 1970). The values of some inorganic constituents in the blood of the camelids have been summarised in table 9, and effect of exercise is shown in Table 10.

Serum iron content is quite variable, i.e. 33 ± 1.32 µg/dl (Soliman and Slaker, 1967) to 110.11 ± 7.07 (65.52-152) µg/dl (Shekhawat *et al.*, 1987). The later workers have also shown the effect of age on iron content, total iron binding capacity (TIBC) and saturation percentage of iron. Serum iron is also affected by pregnancy and it decreases from 91.4 µg/dl in the non-pregnant dromedaries to 64 µg/dl in late pregnancy over seven months. Mean serum copper is about 55.6, 99.7, 47.2 and 86 µg/dl in non-pregnant, mid-pregnancy upto 6 month, late pregnancy over 7 months and puerperium females respectively. Serum zinc content in the corresponding groups was about 58.7, 119.8, 69.1 and 125.9 mg/dl (Elthony *et al.*, 1986).

Table 9. Inorganic constituents of blood in the camelids.

Constituents	Dromedary		Llama[3]	
	Male[1]	Female[2]	Male	Female
Calcium, mg/dl	19.5 ± 8.1	10.8 ± 0.76	8.6 ± 0.5 (7.8-9.7)	9.0 ± 0.5 (7.9-9.8)
Inorganic P, mg/dl	5.6 ± 2.1	6.4 ± 0.41	4.9 ± 1.5 (1.7-7.4)	6.0 ± 2.0 (2.6-9.8)
Magnesium, mg/dl		1.9 ± 0.12		
doo mequi/l			1.9 ± 0.3 (1.5-3.1)	1.9 ± 0.2 (1.5-2.3)
Sodium, mequi/l	17.8 ± 12.7		149 ± 6 (144-168)	152 ± 3 (147-160)
Potassium, mequi/l	2.6 ± 2.2		5.1 ± 1.7 (2.7-7.9)	6.3 ± 0.7 (4.6-7.6)
Sodium chloride, mg/dl		604 ± 4.35		

Sources: 1, Musa & Mukhtar (1982); 2, Soliman & Slaker (1967); 3, Lassen *et al.* (1986).

Table 10. Effect of exercise on inorganic constituents of blood.

Constituents (m.mol/l)	4 km racing Before	After	5 km racing Before	After
Calcium	2.4 ± 0.1	2.5 ± 0.1	2.6 ± 0.1	2.7 ± 0.1
Magnesium	0.76 ± 0.13	0.86 ± 0.15	0.95 ± 0.05	0.04 ± 0.07
Potassium	4.2 ± 0.3	5.1 ± 0.5	4.5 ± 0.3	5.0 ± 0.3
Sodium	154 ± 3.8	158 ± 4.0	154 ± 0.8	158 ± 1.4
Chlorine	116 ± 3.3	118 ± 3.0	116 ± 1.5	117 ± 0.8
Phosphate	2.12 ± 0.23	2.35 ± 0.20	2.24 ± 0.27	2.48 ± 0.25
Bicarbonate	23.6 ± 2.7	10.1 ± 2.8	25.0 ± 1.5	11.6 ± 2.5

Source: Snow *et al.* (1988).

Effect of rut (Musth) on the Haematological changes in male dromedaries.

Some significant differences in the values of white blood cells (WBC) count without any significant effect on the percentage of different leucocytes has been observed during the rut in the male dromedaries of breeding age (Table 11). The fall in haempglobin content is generally due to decreased feed intake and increased aggressiveness in the males during rut period (Khan and Kohli), 1978).

Table 11. Haematology of male camels (Camelus dromedarius) before and during the rut.

Haemogram	Before rut		After rut	
	Range	Mean	Range	Mean
Erythrocytes	7-11.5	8.8	6.5-9.9	8.4
Leucocytes	6.5-13.6	10.5	10.5-19.2	14.16
Lymphocyte, %	43-59	51	47-59	53
Monocyte, %	7-18	13	5-11	7
Neutrophil, %	23-34	27	24-34	29
Eosinophil, %	5-11	9	4-15	9
Basophil, %	1-3	1.9	1-3	1.8
Haemoglobin (g%)	11-14	12.6	9.6-11.8	10.3

References

Abdel-Gadir, S.E., Wahbi, A. and Idris, O.M. 1979. A note on haematology of adult Sudanese camels. Proc. IFS Intern. Symp. on Camels in Sudan, P. 348.

Abdo, M.S., Hassanien, M.M., Manna, M.E. and Hamed, M. 1987. Electrophoretic pattern of serum proteins in the Arabian camel. Indian vet. J., 64: 841.

Adam, S.E.I., Obeid, H.M., Ashour, N. and Tartour, G. 1974. Serum enzyme activities and haematology of normal and diseased ruminants in Sudan. Acta Vet., Brno., 43: 225.

Agar, N.S. and Suzuki, T. 1982. Red cell metabolism in buffaloes and camels. J. Exptl. Zool., 223: 25.

Al-Ali, A.K., Husayni, H.A. and Power, D.M. 1988. A comparative biochemical analysis of the blood of the camel (Camelus dromedarius). Comp. Biochem. Physiol., B, 89: 35.

Alayash, A.I. and Wilson, M.T. 1986. Levels of glycosylated haemoglobin in the Arabian camel (Camelus dromedarius). Comp. Biochem. Physiol., B, 86: 343.

Albritton, E.C. 1952. Standard values in blood. W.B.S. Saunders Co., London.

Aloni, B., Eitan, A. and Livne, A. 1977. The erythrocyte membrane site for the effect of temperature on osmotic fragility. Biochem. Biophysi Acta, 465: 46.

Ateeq, G., Kouider, S. and Kolb, E. 1984. Haematology of dromedaries: cell counts, haemoglobin, proteins, urea, cholesterol, AST and ALT. Age and sex variations. Archiv. fur Exptl. Vet. med., 38: 664.

Ayoub, M.H., Awad, Y.L. and Bayyazeed, L.A. 1960. Calcium level in Egyptian farm animals. Indian J. Vet. Sci. Anim. Husb., 30: 43.

Barakat, M.Z. and Abdel-Fattah, M. 1970. Biochemical analysis of normal camel blood. Zentralbl. Vet. med., 17A, 550.

Bartels, H., Hilpert, P., Barbey, K., Betkey, K., Reigel, K., Lang, E.M. and Metcalfe, J. 1963. Respiratory functions of blood of the yak, llama, camel, Dybowski deer and African elephant. American J. Physiol., 205: 331.

Bhatt, P.L. and Kohli, R.N. 1962. Quantitative biochemical studies on camel's blood. 2. Inorganic phosphorus and sodium content. Indian vet. J., 39: 201.

Chiericato, G.M., Schiappelli, M.P. and abdirahman, A.W. 1986. Characteristics of the blood enzyme and mineral profile of the dromedary (Camelus dromedarius). Clinica Veterinaria, 109, 155.

Cornelius, C.E. and Kaneko, S.J. 1962. Erythrocyte life span in the guanco. Science, 137: 673.

Cornelius, C.E., Kaneko, S.J. 1962. Erythrocyte life span in the guanco. Science, 137: 673.

Eitan, A., Aloni, B. and Livne, A. 1976. Unique properties of the camel erythrocyte membrane. II. Organisation of membrane proteins. Biochem. Biophys. Acta, 426: 647.

Elthony, M.M., Salama, A. and Yousef, A.E.A. 1986. Blood constituents in relation to the reproductive state in she - camel (Camelus dromedarius). Beit. Trop. land, Vet. Med., 24: 425.

Etzoin, Z., Meyerstein, N. and Yagil, R. 1983. Blood sedimentation in the camel. Refuah Vet., 40: 141.

Ghodrian, I., Nowrouzian, I. And Schells, H.F. 1978. A study of some haematological parameters in the Iranian camel. Tropical Anim. Hlth. Prod., 10: 109.

Ghosal, A.K., Alppana, T.C. and Dwaraknath, P.K. 1974. Seasonal variations in water compartments of the Indian camel. British Vet. J., 130, LVii.

Hawkey, C.M. and Gulland, F.M.D. 1988. Haematology of clinically normal and abnormal captive llamas and guanacoes. Vet. Rec., 122: 232.

Jain, N.C. and Keeton, K.S. 1974. orphology of camel and llama erythrocytes as viewed with the scanning electron microscope. British Vet. J., 130: 288.

Kchouk, M. and Durand, M. 1958. Composition of the blood of camel in Tunisia. Arch. Inst. Pasteur, Tunis, 35: 3.

Khan, A.K. and Kohli, I.S. 1978. A note on some haematological studies on male camels (C. dromedarius) before and during rut. Indian J. Anim. Sci., 48: 325.

Kohli, R.N. 1963. Cellular micrometry of camel's blood. Indian vet. J., 40: 134.

Kouider, S., Ateeq, G. and Kolb, E. 1988. Studies on the content of total protein, urea, total fat, cholesterol and bilirubin in blood plasma of camel during the course of a year. Monatshefte fur Vet. med., 43: 139.

Kouider, S. and kolb, E. 1982. Studies into diurnal glucose levels and enzyme activities in serum of camels. Archiv fur Exptl. Vet. med., 36: 601.

Kumar, M., Ghosh, P.K. and De Banerjee, S. 1961. Biochemical stuides on Indian camel (Camelus dromedarius) : Part I - Blood proteins and lipids. J. Sci. Indst. Res., 20C: 236.

Lal, J.B., Bhatt, P.L. and Kohli, R.N. 1962. Quantitative biochemical studies on camel's blood. Part I. Sugar and chloride content. Indian Vet. J., 39: 64.

Lassen, E.D., Pearson, E.G., Long, P., Schmotzer, W.B., Kaneps, A.J. and Riebold, T.W. 1986. Clinical biochemical values of llamas: reference values. American J. Vet. Res., 47: 2278.

Lewis, J.H. 1976. Comparative hematology studies on Camelidae. Comp. Biochem. Physiol., 55A: 367.

Lin, D.K., Bhown, A.S. and Chernoff, A.I. 1976. Studiesnon camel haemoglobin. 1. Physico-chemical properties and some structural aspects of camel haemoglobin (Camelus dromedarius). Biocheimica et Biophysica Acta (P), 434: 110.

Little, A., Mckenzie, A.J., Morris, R.J.H., Roberts, J. and Evans, J.V. 1970. Blood erythrocytes in the Australian camel. Australian J. Exptl. Biol. Med. Sci., 48: 17.

Livne, A. and Kuiper, P.J.C. 1973. Unique properties of the camel erythrocyte membrane. Biochem. Biophys. Acta, 318: 41.

Mohamed, M.H., Mohamed, A.H. and Locatelli, A. 1983. Prolonged water deprivation in the dromedary : effects on plasma proteins and lipoproteins. Vet. Bull. (1985), 55, 215, Abstr. 1723.

Musa, B.E. and Mukhtar, A.M. 1982. Studies on the normal haemogram and some blood electrolytes in camel (Camelus dromedarius). Sudan J. Vet. Sci. Anim. Husb., 23: 38.

Perk, K. 1963. The camel's erythrocytes. Nature, 200: 272.

Perk, K. 1966. Osmotic haemolysis of the camel's erythroagtes. 1. A micro - linematographic study. J. Expt. Zoology, 163: 241.

Per, K., Hort, I., Perri, F. 1963. The degree of swelling and osmotic resistance in hypotonic solutions of erythrocytes from various domestic animals. Refuah Vet., 20: 114.

Ponder, E., yeager, J.F. and Charipper, H.A. 1928. Studies on comparative haematology - camelidae. Q.J. Exp. Physiol., 19: 115.

Rapoport, S. and Guest, G.M. 1941. Distribution of acid-soluble phosphorus in the blood cells of various vertebrates. J. Biol. Chem., 138: 269.

Salib, A.A. and Saleh, S.Y. 1984. Foetal and maternal serum proteins and lactic dehydrogenase during different stages of foetal growth in the camel. Acta Vet., Yogo., 34: 173.

Sharma, D.P., Malik, P.D. and Saprea, K.L. 1973. Age-wise and species-wise haematological studies in farm animals. Indian J. anim. Sci., 43: 289.

Shekhawat, V.S., Bhatia, J.S. and Ghoshal, A.K. 1987. Serum iron and total iron binding capacity in camel. Indian J. Anim. Sci., 57: 168.

Siebert, B.D. and Macfarlane, W.V. 1975. Dehydration in desert cattle and camels. Physiological Zool., 48: 36.

Snow, D.H., Billah, A. and Ridha, A., 1988. effects of maximal exercise on the blood composition of the racing camel. Vet. Rec., 123: 311.

Soliman, M.K. and Slaker, M. 1967. Cytological and biochemical studies on the blood of adult she-camel. Indian vet. J., 44: 989.

Soni, B.K. and Aggarwala, A.C. 1961.

Yagil, R., Sod-Moriah, U.A. and Meyerstein, N. 1974 Dehydration and camel blood. I. Red blood survival in the one-humped camel (Camelus dromedarious). II. Shape, size and concentration of red blood cells. III. Osmotic fragility, specific gravity and osmolality. American J. Physiol., 226, 298, 301, 305.

❑❑❑

Chapter 3

Digestion and Nutrition

Digestive System of the Camelids

The digestive system is one of the important functional system of the body which is mainly responsible for the supply of the nutrients for the maintenance of various body functions. The system is involved right from the selection of feeds to their ingestion, digestion, absorption in the body system, metabolism and elimination of the waste products from the body. The waste products include undigested feed residues and metabolites, and these are mainly eliminated in the form of faeces and urine. The digestive system is a tubulo-muscular canal extending from the buccal cavity to anus. There are several modifications of the digestive tract for the performance of specific functions. The capacious funnel shaped initial part foms the oral cavity. This extends as a narrower tubular structure, the oesophagus which then dilated in different sizes to form compartments 1, 2, 3 and 4 corresponding to the rumen, reticulum, omasum and abomasum of the true ruminants. The intestinal part also has different kinds of sacculation for the formation of caecum and colon. The distal colon is capable to absorb larger proportion of water and forms characteristic faecal pellets. There are some accessory glands like salivary glands, liver and pancreas, which contribute significantly in the digestion of feeds. Since camelids are pseudoruminants, there are ill defined damarcations in the different compartments of the multichambered stomach, while in true ruminants, these are well demarcated (Purohit and Rathore, 1962). There is controversy among the polygastric system of the camelidae. Most of the anatomists as usual like any other ruminant differentiate the compartments of stomach into rumen, reticulum, omasum and abomasum but they also say that histomorphologically these compartments are somewhat different than their counterpart in a true ruminant (Purohit and Rathore, 1962, Vallenas, 1965). The stomach has been differentiated into three compartments by cummings *et al.* (1972). The similarity in the stomach compartments of camel and true ruminants was observed much earlier (Perrault, 1966) and more closer structural similarities were also observed in different species of the camelidae (Droandi, 1936).

Buccal cavity / Mouth

The buccal cavity of camel is formed of the upper jaw, lower jaw, upper bifid lip, lower scoop like conical and pendulous lip and cheeks. The floor of the mouth cavity is formed of dorsal musculo-epithelial surface of the lower jaw. It contains a short, thick and highly mobile tongue. The ceiling is made of a long hard palate and the sides are formed of cheeks. The lips of the camelids are the main organ of prehension and they are highly mobile. these are thin and the upper lip is divided by a median groove or labial cleft. The lower lip is slightly longer, scoop like and pendulous. The upper lip is very sensitive to short out leaves from the thorny plants (Hafez, 1968). The tongue is short, thick and does not protrude. The lamina of the dorsal prominance of the tongue is formed of haline cartilaginous tissue (Vallenas, 1965). The dorsum of the tongue has filiform, fungiform, circum-vallate and a special wart-like papillae. The filiform papillae are conical in shape and have different height and thickness at various levels. The rounded fungiform paillae are surrounded by robust filiform papillae. These are also present on the tip of the ventral surfave of the tongue. These papillae have taste pores on their surfaces. The circumvallate papillae are encircled by a primary groove and an annular pad. The taste pores of these papillae oopen in the grooves. A special type of wart like filiform papillae devoid of taste pores are present on the posterior surface of the tongue (Qayyum *et al.*, 1983). The buccal surface of the cheeks contains long, conical and pigmented papillae of upto 2 cm length. The dental pad is very hard and a pair of incisors and another of canine teeth are also found on the upper jaw. The teeth develop continuously. The masticatory surface of the teeth lacks enamel and has two central invaginations containing both enamel and cement. The adult dromedary had 34 permanent teeth and it may be 36 in some sudanese camels (Leese, 1927). However, New World cameloids had 30 teeth in adult male and 23 in adult female alpaca (Fernandez-Baca, 1961-62). The dental formulae of deciduous (milk) and permanent dentition of dromedary and alpaca are as follows:

i) Dental formulae of Dromedary (common camel)

a) Milk teeth, $I\frac{1}{3}C\frac{1}{1}P\frac{3}{2}M\frac{0}{0}=22$

b) Permanent teeth, $I\frac{1}{3}C\frac{1}{1}P\frac{3}{2}M\frac{3}{3}=34$

for sudanese camel, $I\frac{1}{3}C\frac{1}{3}P\frac{3}{I}M\frac{3}{3}=36$

ii) Dental formulae of Alpaca

a) Milk teeth, $I\frac{0}{3}C\frac{0}{0}P\frac{0}{0}M\frac{3}{3}=16$

b) Permanent teeth in male, $I\frac{1}{3}C\frac{1}{1}P\frac{2}{1}M\frac{3}{3}=30$

c) Permanent teeth in female, $I\frac{1}{3}C\frac{1}{1}P\frac{2}{1}M\frac{2}{3}=28$

The use of dentition and eruption pattern for the estimation of age of the camelidae has been reported in dromedary (Leese, 1927, Acland, 1932, Williamson and Payne, 1978). The central pair of incisors is already present at birth and by one month second pair and two months third pair erupts. The teeth are crowned and begins wearing at about one year of age and by two years they do not touch each other due to significant wearing. At about 4 years of age, the teeth are completely worn out and loose with square or irregular table. At about 5 years of age, the central pair of permanent teeth erupts. This is followed by the second pair at about 6 years and third pair at about 7 years of age.

Pharynx

The parynx is a long and narrow passage. It may be divided into an anterior and a posterior compartment due to the presence of a transverse mucosal fold. The anterior compartment is sac like and provides favourable place for the development of the camel bots (Cephalomyia larvae).

Oesphagus

The oesophagus is a long and capacious musculo-epiuthelial tube, which is a continuation of the pharynx terminating into the rumen. The length of oesophagus depends on the size of the animal and may be 1-2 m long. The luminal mucosa of oesophagus is lined by glands which secrete mucous. This helps in the easy passage of feed bolus and provides protection against the injury due to eating of coarse and thorny forages.

Salivary glands

The Salivary glands of the camelids are somewhat similar to those of cattle. These are a pair of well-developed parotid, inferior molar, submaxillary and less developed sublingual glands. Some minute salivary glands have also been reported at the base of the cheek papillae (Leese, 1927). The average weight of the fresh salivary glands in the dromedary of 200-300 kg body weight has been found to be about 116, 24, 41 and 4 g for the both parotids, molar, submaxillary and sublingual glands respectively. Sheets of small mucous glands are formed on the cheeks and palates. The parotid and inferior molar glands are purely serous glands while others are the muco-serous glands (Hoppe *et al.,* 1975).

Complex chambered stomach system

Like true ruminants, the camelids also possess multichambered polygastric system. There is difference of opinion among the researchers regarding the number of the compartments in the stomach of the camelids. This is due to lack of well-defined demarcation between the third and fourth compartments. A few workers (Leonard, 1891, Leese, 1927, Purohit and Rathore, 1962) dfferentiated compartmental stomach system of the camels into four chambers corresponding to the rumen, reticulum, omasum and abmasum of the cattle, while some others preserred to differentiate into only three chambers, viz. compartment 1 (rumen or C1), compartment 2 (Reticulum or C2) and compartment 3 (abomasum or C3) or true stomach (Vallenas *et al.,* 1971, Heller *et al.,* 1986) in the alpaca and llamas. The absence of true omasum has also been described in the dromedary (Mohammed, 1979). In the present chapter, the stomach system of camelids has been described as a four chambered polygastric system comprising of less developed rumen, reticulum, omasum and abomasum considering the camelids as a stage earlier than the ruminants in the evolution process or a modified system for a different herbage feeding cleass of animals. Since the glandular ruminal sacs, reticulum and omasum are lined with the simple columnar epithelium, they can not be considered as proventriculus or oesophageal sacculations.

Rumen or Compartment C1

The rumen is the largest chamber of the polygastric system. It is different from the rumen of cattle due to the presence of two, i.e. one anterior and another posterior sac. These sacs were initially considered as chambers ots for water storage in camels, which is not true (Leonard, 1891). However, Leese (1927) regarded these sacs as the collection of deep cells for the storage of water.

The rumen in Bikaneri camels extends from the posterior border of the eighth rib to the transverse process of the last lumber vertebra (Purohit and Rathore, 1962). It occupies larger part of the left abdominal cavity and extends over the median plane ventrally. The parietal (left) surface of rumen is placed along the diaphragm, left wall of the abdominal cavity and the spleen. The visceral (right) surface is related to the surfaces of reticulum, omasum, abomasum, liver, intestines, right kidney and pancreas. The dorsal curvature is in contact with the visceral surface of the first four lumbar vertebrae and the ventral curvature lies on the floor of the abdomen. The grooves on the outer surface of the rumen are quite faint and it is difficult to differentiate the rumen into dorsal ventral sacs. The rumen does not contain well defined muscular pillars and its mucous membrane is not studded with papillae. However, at certain places the ruminal mucosa is raised into small rounded points, which are more prominent in its centre. The remaining mucous membrane is smooth. The interior surface is lined with squamous epithelium except its glandular sac region which is lined by the simple columnar epithelium.

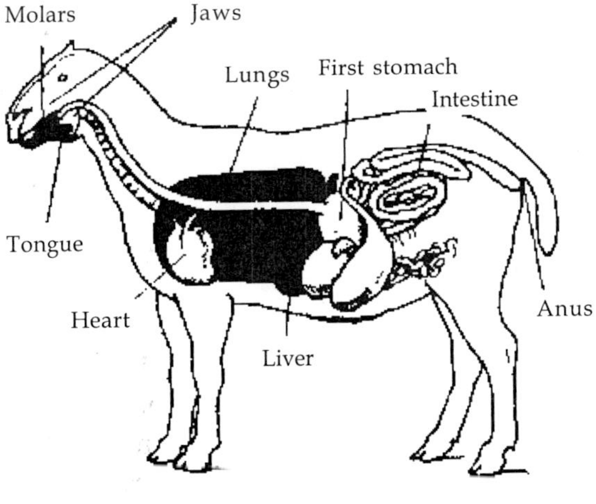

Fig. 1. Digestive System of camel

In case of alpaca (Lama pacos), however, the rumen has been differentiated into the dorsal and ventral sacs by a muscular fold running from the cordiac entrance to the posterior third of the rumen. The presence of 13-15 grooves anteriorly and ventral to the muscular fold has been observed. These grooves are separated by ridges formed at right angles and parallel to the muscular fold, which from 3 to 10 pouches of varying size in each groove. The irregular bottom surface of these pouches is due to the folds in the mucosa. The orifices of the pouches are constricted by the membranous folds inserted into the ridges. The dorsal sac is further divided into two portions. Out of these, one portion is again divided by several oblique grooves and contains variable number of pouches. The other portion is free from the grooves and pouches. The dorsal sac is more thick and surface mucosa is thinner and covered with smooth mucosa. The lamina propria contains small mucous type glands formed by a single layer of cells on a basal membrane. The glandular epithelium is almost in line with the mucosa and the glands open into the lumen of the pouches (Vallenas, 1965).

The glandular sacs of the rumen of dromedary: Unlike true ruminants in the camelids two special small compartments are present on the antero-inferior and medio-inferior aspect of the rumen. These are separated from the main ruminal cavity by strong muscular folds. The antero-inferior sac is more on the right side communicating with the reticulum and the medio-inferior sac lies on the floor of the abdominal cavity. The interior surface of these glandular sacs is formed of smaller compartments divided by strong longitudinal bands. Most of these compartments are further divided by the transverse bands which gives them honeycomb like appearance. Due to this structure, the antero-inferior sac may be confused with the reticulum. The longitudinal bands of the antro-inferior glandular sac have stouter muscular bands than those of the medio-inferior sac. The transverse bands are thinner and much less in number. On the other hand, the pouches in the medio-inferior glandular sac are deeper than those of the antero-inferior glandular sac and a few of them are also not partitioned by the transverse bands. In the walls of these glandular sacs, two sets of parallel muscular bundles arranged at right angles to each other are present. The glandular sacs are lined by simple columnar epithelium above their bottoms and contain tubular glands. Microscopically these are similar to large intestine except that the crypts are shallow and the goblet cells are few in number (Purohit and Rathore, 1962, Schmidt-Nielsen, 1964).

Reticulum

The reticulum of the camelids is small and pear shaped or kidney shaped and appears to be in continuation with the antero-inferior glandular sac of the rumen, posteriorly. It is situated on the right of the median plane and it communicates anteriorly with the omasum. The paretal surfaces is placed along the liver and visceral surface is in contact with the right aspect of the rumen.

The interior surface of the reticulum contains many deep pouches separated from each other by muscular bands numbering 11-15 and directed towards the oesophageal groove (Leonard, 1891, Purohit and Rathor, 1962, Vallenas, 1965). Each pouch is again divided and sub-divided to form smaller cells resembling the honeycomb. The uppermost cells of these pouches are either square or rectangular and arranged in about 12 parallel rows in the Bikaneri camel. The mucosa of these pouches is studded with very small rounded papillae and the mucous membrane is lined with simple columnar epithelium (Purohit and Rathore, 1962). There are also tubular mucous type glands in the epithelium. The oesophageal groove is more or less similar to the ruminants and continues from the cordiac orifice to the entrance of the omasum or third compartment of the four compartment classification.

Omasum

The omasum begins as a narrow musculo-tubular extension of the reticulum, which is elongated and caudally becomes uniform in diameter. The reticulo-omasal junction is situated on the left side of the abdominal cavity but the greater part of the omasum lies on the right side, where it is almost covered by the liver. The visceral surface is related to the rumen wall. The mucous membrane is folded and about 50 longitudinal folds give a leafy appearance. The folds do not run throughout the length of the omasum and each fold obliterates on the way and gives rise to another fold to cover the remaining part. The folds are thinner and narrower than in the cattle and non-papillated. The muscular portion of the omasum possesses transverse bands of smooth muscle fibres (Purohit and Rathore, 1962). In the alpaca, the omasum has been found to be continuous with the abomasums without any sphincter or narrow band separating the two compartments (Vallenas, 1965). However, in the dromedary presence of one sided constriction in the middle of the omasum has been reported (Leese, 1927). A true omasum is, however, absent in the dromedary (Mohammed, 1979) and also in other camelids.

Abomasum or True stomach

The abomasum in camelids is similar to other ruminants and it is related to the rumen, reticulum and omasum. External demarcation between omasum and abomasum is not distinct (Leese, 1927, Purohit and Rathore, 1962). Internally the abomasum is divided into two regions, the anterior fundic and posterior pyloric part. The mucous membrane of the fundic part possesses distinct rounded laminae, which are connected at bottom with each other by thick folds of mucous membrane numbering about 17. The middle folds are thicker and larger. The pyloric mucosa is plain but may contain a few distinct folds. The internal surface is lined with simple columnar epithelium (Purohit and Rathore, 1962). The average thickness of the pyloric mucosa is about 1243 μm anteriorly which gradually decreases to 1064 μm in the middle pyloric region of the abomasum of dromedary (Dougbag and Berg, 1981). The abomasum has also been described to be somewhat similar to the stomach of the swine (Mohammed, 1979).

The glandular mucosa in the polygastric system of camelids

The glandular mucosa in all the compartments of the complex stomach of llama was recognized (Brandt, 1841), which was subsequently described in the dromedary (Pilliet, 1885). Many observers noted the resemblance of the glandular mucosa with the cordiac gland mucosa (Hansen and Schmidt-Nielsen, 1957, Moir, 1968).

Descriptive observations on the complex stomach of the dromedary, llama and guanaco revealed that all the compartments of the stomach system possess mucilagenous glandular mucosa. The interior of the dorsal parts of the compartment 1 and 2, viz, the rumen and reticulum are lined with a smooth layer of the stratified squamous epithelium without papillae, whereas the ventral parts of all the compartments of the complex stomach are lined with glandular mucosa (Dellmann *et al.*, 1968, Cummings *et al.*, 1972, Luciano *et al.*, 1979). This mucosa lined the recessed saccules of the first compartment or rumen, the deep cells of the second compartment (reticulum) and the anterior 80 per cent portion of the combined third compartment (omaso-abomasum). The non-recessed area of the first compartment is covered by the stratified squamous epithelium, which also includes the crests defining the individual glandular saccules. This also covered the gastric groove as it extended along the lesser curvature of the second compartment and terminated as a narrow tubular passage to the third compartment. In the terminal 20 per cent portion of the combined third compartment the usual gastric and pyloric glands are present.

The mucigenous glandular mucosa is folded in the saccules of the first compartment and papillated in the cells of the second compartment. It is arranged in a retiform in the one-fifth portion of the third compartment and in the middle three-fifth portion, is formed permanent longitudinal folds. There is no difference in the structure of the mucigenous glandular mucosa due to its different arrangements in the various parts of the complex stomach. The tall columnar cells on the luminal surface continued into the shallow foveola. Each foveola tapered deep and it was continuous through an isthmus with a short end piece of gland. Sometimes end pieces penetrated through the muscularis mucosae reaching the submucosa.

Cytologically the epithelium of mucous membrane may be differentiated into four regions, viz. the luminal surface epithelium, the foveolar epithelium, the isthemic epithelium and the epithelium of end-piece ot tail-piece. The luminal surface epithelium covers the ridges between the faveolae. The faveolar epithelium covers the short funnel shaped gastric pits. The isthemie epithelium lines the narrow junctional length connecting the deep parts of the foveola and the gland's end-piece, and the short slightly expanded terminal portion of the gland tubule is lined with the cells of the end-piece (Cummings *et al.,* 1972). The luminal surface epithelium is formed of laterally compressed tall cells containing mucous granules. The concentration of the mucous granules increases in the cells nearer to the foveolar orifice, and they are maximum in the foveolar epithelium where almost half of the cells contain mucous granules. Many endocrine cells are also found in this region (Rubsamen and Engelhardt, 1979, Luciano *et al.,* 1980).

Epithelium of the gland isthmus

Although it is often not easy to deliniate the isthmus precisely in a gland, it is either equal or exceeds the end-piece in length. This region is easily identified by the presence of mitotic division and frequently 3 to 4 dividing cells may be seen in a section of a single isthmus. The interphase cells of this region are short (about 12 μ) and pyramidal. Each cell contains a basally placed large and spherical nucleus. On staining with haematoxalin and eosin the perinuclear region stains basophilically while the supranuclear cytoplasm more lightly with eosin (Cumming *et al.,* 1972).

Epithelium of the gland end-piece

The epithelial cells of the end-piece are pyramidal in shape and slightly shorter (9u) than the cells of the isthmus. The nuclei are basally placed and appears compressed in the cells at the blind end of the tubule. The supranuclear region appears to be covered by a pale vesicular mass. This is most heavily accumulated in the cells at the blind end of the tubules and clearly exceeds to that found in the cells of the isthmus. The cells closer to the isthmus are intermediary in density in the vesicular supranuclear region (Cumming *et al.*, 1972).

Foveolar epithelium

The height of foveolar cells progressively increases from the isthmus towards the foveolar orifice. The cells near the orifice of foveola are 18 to 19 μ, whereas deeper one are 14 to 15 μ in height. An oval nucleus is situated at the base of the cells. The perinuclear region appears slightly baso-philic, while supranuclear region contains a large pale vesicular mass which is largest in the cells of upper part of the foveola. The apical aspect of the vesicular mass is delimited by a granular eosinophilic substance, which is covered by a narrow pale zone (Cumming *et al.*, 1972).

Epithelium of the luminal surface

The surface cells of the lumen in the region of foveolar orifice resemble the foveolar cells. This resemblance in cells diminishes progressively with the increase in the distance from the foveola. The surface epithelial cells are taller and narrower than the cell in the upper region of the foveola. These surface cells possess numerous apical microvilli. Apically the adjacent cell surfaces are relatively straight and closely levelled. On moving more baselly, long microvillus processes are seen and the intercellular space is often very prominent.

The supranuclear accumulations of the mitochondria increases gradually at increasing distance from the foveola. This is associated with a corresponding reduction in mucogen granules. The mitochondria corresponds in location with the eosinophilic material covering much of the supranuclear region. In addition to these, there are also degenerated surface cells, which are normally found at some distance from the foveolar orifice. These cells contain a small centrally placed nucleus, electron lucent cytoplasm, relatively few organelles and few or no mucigen granules. The apical micro villi are absent and the junctional complexes and desmosomes, which join the more viable surface cells, are not observed. Some mitochondria persisted in the supranuclear cytoplasm. The profiles of granular reticulum and the Golgi complex were also recognizable. Some of the degenerating cells contain cytoplasmic dense bodies and a few cells may be partially extruded from the adjacent cells (Cumming *et al.*, 1972).

Pyloric mucosa

The pyloric mucosa is foldless. Average thickness of mucosa in initial part is about 1243 μm,which gradually decreases to 1064 μm in the mid-pyloric region (Dougbag and Berg, 1981).

Capacity of different compartments of camelid's stomach

The average volume of the rumen of the Bikaneri camel is 50-90 litres (Purohit and Rathore, 1962). The contents of the first two compartments (rumen and reticulum) of the camel's stomach is about 10-15 per cent of the body weight (Engelhardt and Rubsamen, 1979). Further 1-2 per cent is hold by the third compartment (Rubsamen, 1978). Average 6.5 pH in the omasum drops much below pH 4 in the abomasum. The various epithelial cells of the abomasum viz., the mucous cells, parietal cells, chief cells and endocrine cells are almost similar to those found in the stomach of the monogastric animals (Lucian and Engelhardt, 1980). The pH of abomasal content of the camel averaging 3.6 is higher than the pH 2.3 in zebu cattle kept under similar conditions of feeding (Maloiy, 1972).

Intestines

The intestines are as usual differentiated into the duodenum, ileum, jejunum, caecum, colon and rectum. The length of small intestine is about 4 meters and common bile duct and pancreatic duct opens into the duodenum at about a distance of half meter from the pylorus (Leese, 1927). The gall bladder is absent in the camelids.

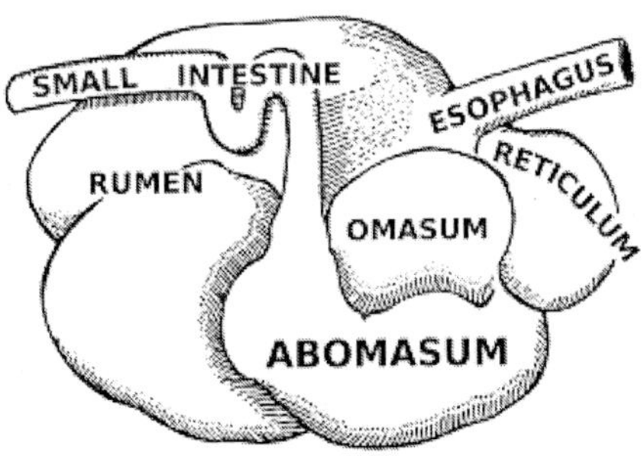

Fig. 2 : Stomach of Camel

Most of the jejunum is placed in the right portion of the abdominal cavity and a chain of mesentric lymph nodes are linked with the duodenum. Another series of mesentric lymph nodes surround the anterior mesentric arteries. The lymphatics of the distal pert of the ileum also drain the colon. The length of the colon is about 19-20 meters, which is larger proximally and coiled like that in swine distally. The caecum is comparable to that of cattle.

Liver

The liver of the camelids is highly lobulated and does not contain a gall bladder. Therefore, there is no storage of bile in the camelids. The right lobe is largest and forms more than half of the organ. The surface of the liver is engraved by a large number of small fissures (Ouhsine and Zguigal, 1983). The bile duct joins the pancreatic duct to drain through a common duct into the duodenum.

Pancreas

The pancreas is a flattened quadrilateral organ containing a long left and a short right lobe. The major pancreatic duct is formed of branches from the both lobes of the pancreas and subsequently joins the hepatic duct. The minor pancreatic duct is not found. The blood is supplied through the branches from the nepatic and cranial mesentric arteries and drains to the portal vein. The major splanchnic nerve supplies the sympathetic nerve branches while vagus supplies the parasympathetic fibres (Mostafa *et al.*, 1982a, b).

Spleen

The spleen of bactrian and dromedary camels is large weighing 5 to 7 kg in adults. In llamoids, it is generally less than 1 kg weight in most of the animals.

Functions of the digestive system

The digestive system is responsible for the supply of nutrients for supporting various physiological functions of animals. Main functions of the digestive system may be listed as follows:

1. Identification and selection of feeds - Under natural habitat, the camelids are free to find their feeds and water needs from the herbages and water sources on the grass lands and ranges. The dromedaries are mainly found in the hot deserts, whereas

bactrians belong to cold deserts. The herbage cover is generally scarce. Mostly herbs, shrubs and thorny trees are found scarcely distributed on the arid lands of the Indian subcontinent and Africa. The situation in semi-arid region and riverine areas is somewhat better. The camels are frequently required to walk long distances in search of feed and water. Practice of camping near a water source is a common practice of camel rearing in the pastoralist groups.

2. Eating and storage of feeds - Long, bifid and mobile upper lip assisted by tongue and incisor teeth are responsible for the holding and biting of herbages. After few chewings, the feeds are ingested and stored in the rumen, which are further masticated during rumination for providing larger area for the action of microbes and their enzymes. The ingested feeds are mixed with saliva and degraded rumen contents including the ruminal micro-organisms.

3. Rejection of harmful materials - The bifid upper lip, a pair of upper incisors and long papillae in the mouth cavity help camels to short out thorns, spines and other extraneous materials. The off flavour and unwanted taste are the other factors for discarding the feeds. Sometimes harmful materials are ingested inadvertently or due to lack of differentiation. Such substances are rapidly expelled out by increasing the rate of passage and exosmosis causing diarrhoea by drawing water from the body and increasing the peristalsis.

4. Digestion, absorption and metabolism of feeds – In the camels digestion of feeds is microbial as in true ruminants in the first and second compartments. Anaerobic micro-organisms in the first compartment or rumen are capable to ferment the fibrous feeds into volatile fatty acids (VFA), synthesize amino acids and proteins from the non-protein nitrogenous (NPN) compounds and synthesize almost all kinds of water soluble vitamins.

5. Transportation of the nutrients across the walls of the alimentary canal - The simpler compounds of smaller molecular weight formed during the microbial and enzymic digestion in different segments of the digestive system are absorbed into the body system by active and selective absorption and also by passive diffusion. The absorbed nutrients are carried to liver and tissues by the circulatory and lymphatic systems. Liver is the main site of metabolism as well as storage of the nutrients.

pungens, about 40 per cent visited water source at 5 days interval, 30 per cent after 4 days, 20 per cent after 6 days and 10 per cent after 7 days in the month of July in north-west Sahara (Gauthier-Pilters, 1972). About 1-20 g feed is eaten in each bite depending on the leafyness of the herbages and mouth is full after several bites. The small bites are plucked from the thorny plants, twigs containing few scattered leaves, dry grasses and small plants. The camels do not close their mouth on eating the thorny plants. The herbages collected in the mouth is chewed slowly and thoroughly (Gauthier-Pilters and Dagg, 1981). The camels browse for 5-20 minutes at a stretch end, then chew for 10-15 minutes for regurgitation. The cycle is repeated during the grazing period. The rate of grazing and regurgitation decreases as the day progresses and it becomes very slow in the afternoon between 6-8 p.m.

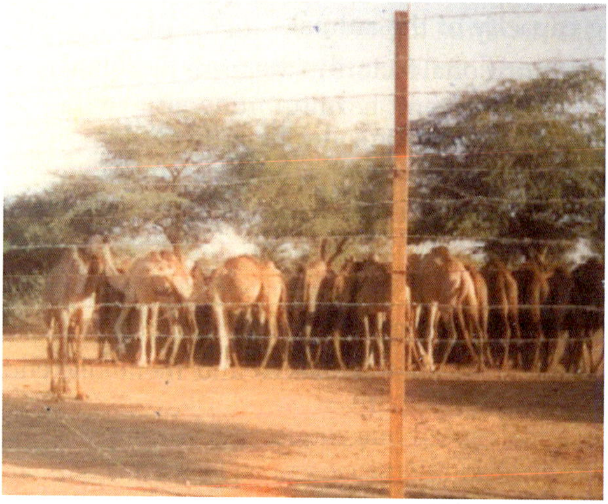

Camels browsing acacia

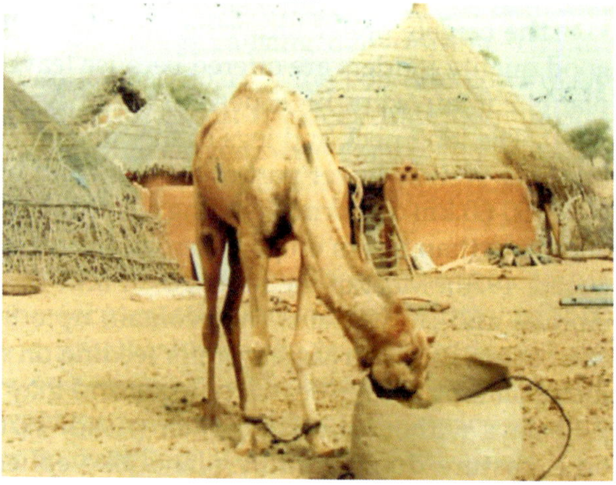

Camel feeding on stall

(Anonymous, 1992-93). Such changes in feeding behaviour might be due to attainment of satiety and/or fatigue of the jaw muscles. Each bolus is chewed for 40-50 times before regurgitation. The camels chew on one side at a time by changing side in alternate chewing (Mcfarlane, 1964).

Selection of feeds on range land

The camels feed selectively and often avoid grazing on dense and succulent vegetation and wove to drier plants discarded by other grazing species (Gauthier-Pilters and Dagg,1981). This is contrary to the other observations where preference for thorny and salty plants containing about 80 per cent water has been shown (Mcfarlane, 1964). Average moisture percentage in some plants eaten by the camels ranged from 58-88 (Table 12) and almost all species contained higher than 13 per cent crude protein and high level of energy on dry matter basis (Maloiy, 1972).

Table 12. Moisture, crude protein and energy values of plants.

Name of plant	Moisture (%)	Crude protein (%)	Gross energy (Kcal/kg DM)
Acacia brevispica	58	17.75	3958
do (green pods)	74	23.45	6720
A. mellifera	65	18.44	4472
A. senegalensis	67	13.00	4027
A. tortilis	64	19.62	4550
Capitanya spp.	88	16.25	4007
Duosperma eremophilum	73	16.63	2746
Kleinia spp.	78	7.25	4385

Voluntary feed intake

Limited informations are available on the voluntary feed intake of camels because of the difficulties in determination of feed intake on browses. On most of the pastures, the camels consume 10-20 kg green fodders supplying about 5-10 kg dry matter but on succulent herbages feed intake may be 30-40 kg providing 6-8 kg dry matter. However, adult camels may be maintained on the feeding of 3-5 kg dry matter per day from relatively low grade dry fodders (Gauthier-Pilters and Dagg, 1981).

Like other animals the voluntary feed intake in camels is significantly influenced by several factors like nature of the feeds, physiological state of the animal and dehydration, etc. The palatability of dub (Cynodon dactylon) hay is low in camels and voluntary intake has been observed to be 3.2 ± 0.2 kg per day on ad libitum feeding in adult camels (Maloiy, 1972). Moth (Phaseolus aconitifolia) fodder is highly palatable and its average daily intake has been found to be 9.5 ± 0.95 kg on sole feeding and 11.45 ± 1.75 kg, when it is supplemented with 2.25 kg concentrates (Bhatia *et al.*, 1998). Similarly, mean intake of moth fodder, dry empty pods of clustter bean (guar) and gram straw has been found to be about 112 ± 13, 83 + 4 and 77 ± 5 g per kg W 0.75 (metabolic body weight) respectively on ad libitum feeding. Voluntary feed intake in lactating females 8.78 ± 0.16 kg has been found to be much higher than 6.13 ± 0.61 kg eaten by dry females (Jakhmola, 1992-93). Dehydration has adverse effect on voluntary feed intake and decrease in feed intake depends on the degree and duration of dehydration. An average 15.06 ± 0.55 g dry matter intake per kg body weight in hydrated camels drastically reduced to only 2.27 ± 0.52 g per kg body weight after 3 days of dehydration in Bikaneri camels and became negligible from the fourth day of dehydration. However, recovery in feed intake was faster on rehydration and it increased to 6.99 ± 1.97 g per kg body weight within 72 hours of rehydration (Anonymous, 1992-93). Average diet of the pastoral camels in Kenya is made of predominantly dwarf shrubs followed by trees, grasses, other herbs and vines constituting about 48, 30, 11,10 and 1 per cent of total intake respectively (Field, 1979). However, considerable variation may be observed between dry and wet season.

Salivary Secretion

Copious secretion from the salivary glands in the camelids is almost a continuous process. The parotid and inferior molar glands are exclusive serous, while others are muco-serous glands. Larger amount of saliva is secreted by the parotid glands. A daily flow of about 21 litre saliva from one parotid gland has been reported in the adult dromedary but variation is quite high which is affected by several factors like feeding, dehydration and species (Table 13). Flow rate of saliva in dromedaries (Hoppes *et al.*, 1974, Bhatia *et al.*, 1986) has been found to be higher than the flow rate in alpaca (Ortiz *et al.*, 1974). The values of pH and some ionic constituents of parotid saliva of dromedary and alpaca (Table 14) show little variation which may be due to differences in the nature of feeds or other factors. Amylase activity has been reported in the parotid saliva of dromedary (Mura *et al.*, 1983) but such activity in bovine saliva once reported in the saliva was later found to be secreted from the nasolabial glands (Church, 1988).

Table 13. Flow rate of saliva in dromedary and alpaca.

Particulars	Dromedary*		Alpaca**
	Range	Mean	Mean
Saliva flow (ml/h)	385-499	443 ± 13.3	
before feeding	428-457	447 ± 9.3	140 ± 5.6
during feeding	360-650	482 ± 35.4	202 ± 15.1
post feeding	250-480	315 ± 23.7	159 ± 15.0
in night (rest)	492-518	502 ± 8.7	not recorded
Total/gland/day (1)	9.2-11.7	10.6 ± 0.3	-

NB: *Bhatia *et al.*, 1986; **Ortiz *et al.*, 1974

Table 14. The values of pH and composition of parotid saliva of dromedary and alpaca.

Constituents of saliva	Arabian dromedary[1]		Indian dromedary[2]	Alpaca[3]
	Dehydrated	Hydrated	Hydrated	Normal
Volume/gland/day (1)	3.0	15.0	10.6	-
Specific gravity	-	-	1.0108	-
pH	-	-	8.06 – 8.23	8.6
Ions (mequi/l),				
Sodium	202	162	173 ± 3.4	165–172
Potassium	4	24	11.5 ± 0.12	9.4–13.7
Magnesium	-	-	0.8 ± 0.05	-
Bicarbonates	112	119	100 ± 3.25	121–128
Phosphates	30	8	18.3 ± 1.02	31–34
Chlorides	38	16	20.9 ± 0.35	-

Sources: 1, Hoppes *et al.*, 1974; 2, Bhatia *et al.*, 1986; 3, Ortiz *et al.*, 1974.

Rumen motility and passage of digesta

Through the digestive tract of the camelids

The motility of forestomach, retention time of digesta in the compartments 1 and 2 (rumen and reticulum) and rate of passage of digesta through the digestive tract have been studied in the dromedary (Maloiy, 1972, Heller *et al.*, 1986, Bhatia *et al.*, 1988) and llamoids (Vallenas, 1965, Vallenas and Stevens, 1971). The motility pattern in all the camelids is more or less similar except the number of movements and the intensity of contraction which differ between the species and also influenced by the composition of diets and the extent of dehydration.

A cyclic pattern of motility occurs in compartment 1 and 2 of the forestomach which are called A and B contractions. Mean motility cycle in dromedary is composed of 7 A and 5 B cycles in 5 minutes including a pause of about 2.3 minutes (Heller *et al.*, 1986). A single rapid contraction of the reticulum or compartment 2 (C2) initiates the motility cycle. This is quickly followed by simultaneous contraction of both sacs, i.e. caudo-dorsal and caudo-ventral region of the rumen or compartment 1 (Cl) and then by the contraction of its crania sac. The first set of contractions of the caudal and cranial region of Cl is followed by series of 6-8 additional contractions before the contraction of C2. The amplitude of contraction of C1 during each cycle is increased and then decreased with the progress of the cycle. The last caudal sac contraction in a cycle is not followed by a corresponding contraction of cranial region which always shows one contraction less than the caudal sac. The last contraction of caudal sac is followed by a pause in the contraction of C1 until C2 contracted again to initiate another cycle.

The duration of a cycle, the period of time between C2 is 1.8 + 0.2 minutes in the resting llama. The feeding has non-significant effect on the contraction of C2, but there is marked and significant increase in contractions of C1 after feeding. The amplitude of all contractions increases. The contractions return to resting stage within 20 minutes of stopping feeding. After about 20 minutes, again the amplitude of caudal sac contractions increases and remains significantly higher for 80-100 minutes after feeding. The amplitudes of cranial sac of Cl and C2 start to diminish to the pre-feeding levels immediately upon removal of feeds and there is no significant difference 40 minutes post-feeding. The mean duration of a cycle in the resting llama is 1.8 + 0.2 minutes (Vallenas, 1965) and in dromedary 1-2 minutes (Engelhardt and Rubsamen, 1979).

During contraction of C2, the contents are pushed into the caudal sac of Cl. On the contraction of caudal sac, some of the contents enters into the cranial sac and rest returns back into C2. The final contraction of cranial sac passes back the ingesta into the caudal sac (Ehrlein and Engelhardt, 1971). During the process, the contents of the dorsal sac rotate anticlockwise and fluid is sqeezed out due to strong contractions. This activity and more frequent cycle of rumination combined with glandular pouch secretions may provide for more mixing, maceration and buffering of digesta causing greater efficiency of digestion (Vallenas and Stevens, 1971). The proximal portion of the less defined compartment 3 (C3) contracts before the first strong contraction of C2. After the entrance of digesta in C3, the proximal portion contracts and the distal portion dilates. The Contractions are more pronounced in the distal portion of C3 and it may be defined as peristaltic in nature (Ehrlein and Engelhardt, 1971). Rumination starts with the greatest contraction of the cranial sac of C1 and may be 3-4 times per cycle.

Eructation takes place near the peak of a caudo-dorsal and ventral sac contraction 3-4 times per cycle. It is not linked with the contraction of cranial sac or C2. Abdominal pressure does not appear to be associated with the eructation which is usually immediately followed by deglutition. Deglutition may be observed at any stage of the cycle.

During the process of rumination, the cranial sac shows extra contractions which are not preceded by the contractions of the caudal sac. These contractions are accompained by regurgitation. The contractions of C2 are totally unrelated to regurgitation and 3-4 regurgitations may occur in a single motility cycle. An average 7 rumination cycles per 5 minutes are observed in the llamids.

The motility of abomasum is somewhat different than the forestomach. The contractions of proximal part are of small amplitude while those of distal part show an increase of pressure of greater amplitude and duration during each cycle. The pressure wave is preceded by a single drop in pressure at the time of contraction of C2 and interrupted by small negative pressure waves which coincide with contractions of the caudal sac of C1 (Vallenas and Stevens, 1971).

The rotention time feeds in the forestomach is as usual influenced by several factors like nature of diet, composition of diet and water intake. Mean retention time of feeds in the forestomach is 46 to 50 hours under different conditions (Maloiy, 1972, Bhatia *et al.*, 1988). The retention of fluid and particles in the digestive tract of the llama has been found to 15.3 + 3.1, 27.0 + 4.4 and 32.5 + 5.7 hours for fluid, small particles and large particles respectively. The retention time of fluid, small particles of 2-10 mm and larger particles of 2.5-4.0 cm in C1 (rumen) is about 9.7, 19.2 and 25.0 hours; and whole digestive tract is about 36.2 ± 6.0, 52.0 ± 5.3 and 59.9 ± 6.2 hours, repectively (Heller *et al.*, 1986b). A detail account of rate of passage in dromedary on the feeding of two diets (Table 15) shows some variations (Bhetia *et al.*, 1988). On the feeding of same fodder the feed retention time in dromedary, 46 ± 0.84 hours was mach less than 55 ± 0.74 hours in the zebu cattle. This resulted into lower dry matter digestibility in camel than the zebu cattle (Maloiy, 1972).

Table 15. Rate of passage of digesta throught the digestive tract of dromedary camel on two diets.

Particulars	Diet 1	Diet 2
Phaseolus aconitifolia (moth) fodder	Fed	Fed
Concentrate pellets	Fed	Not fed
Dry matter intake/day (kg)	11.45 ± 1.75	9.50 ± 0.95
Moisture % in faeces	70.74 ± 2.84	68.86 ± 3.79
Excretion started (h) after feeding	16	18
5 % Excretion time (h)	19.93 ± 1.26	21.21 ± 0.87
95 % Excretion time (h)	78.33 ± 4.91	80.58 ± 3.76
5-95% Excretion time (h)	58.40	59.37
Mean retention time (h)	47.32 ± 1.74	50.18 ± 1.72

Significantly higher digestibility of alfalfa hay and pelleted ration in llamoids in comparison to sheep and pony may be considered due to longer retention time in the llamoids (Hintz *et al.*, 1978).

Rumen contents

The capacity of rumen dromedary may be higher than 100 litres (Purohit and Rathor, 1963). Dromedaries drink 100-135 litres water at a time but under dehydrated condition, the amount of water drinking may be upto 200 liters in a camel of about 600 kg body weight (Gauthier-Pilters, 1972, Yagil *et al.*, 1974). However, solids constitute less than 15 per cent under normal conditions. The capacity of rumen in llamoids is 10-15 liters. Llamoids replace about 67 per cent water loss by drinking water in about 8 minutes, then they may replace the remaining deficit grdually in about 2 days time (Macfarlane, 1964). Thus, the llamoids are not as fast drinkers as the dromedary.

Average volume of rumen contents is 45-48 litres in the dromedary (Maloiy, 1972) and about 10 litres in adult llama (Vellenas and Stevens,

1971). Total stomach and intestina1 fill in adùlt male dromedary is about 78 kg and in females 88 kg which are about 16.8 and 21.3 per cent of the body weight respectively (Wilson, 1978). The fermentation pattern in the rumen of the camelids is more or less similar to the true ruminants except that substantial amount of lactic acid is also produced in addition to volatile fatty acids (VFA) which may be 9.32-65.20 mg per cent (mean 33.21 mg %) of the rumen liquor (Ghosal *et al.*, 1981). Total VFA content in the rumen liquor of camelids may vary from 80-150 mequi per litre depending on the feed and water supply (Anonymous, 1971, Maloiy, 1972, Ghosal *et al.*, 1981). The VFA content is also significantly affected by the pH of rumen contents and it has been observed to be about 90, 135 and 150 mequi per litre at pH 6.5, 6.0 and 5.8 respectively (Maloiy, 1972). The concentration of VFA also differs in the contents of Cl, C2 and C3 compartments. Substantial amount of VFA is also present in the caecum and colon of the camelids indicating active microbial activities in these segments. An average 129, 116, 88.6, 74.7, 66.0, 19.9, 9.4, 11.6, 39.7 and 57.1. m mol per litre VFA concentration has been reported in the contents of proximal C1, distal C1, C2, proximal C3, middle C3, distal C3, duodenum, ileum, caecum and colon respectively (Anonymous, 1971). The percentage of acetic, propionic, butyric and valeric acid in total VFA of rumen in dromedary has been found to be about 57.65 (50-63.4), 18.05 (16.6-19.92), 32.25 (30.0-33.11) and 1.22 (traces to 1.3) per cent respectively. The values of total nitrogen, amonia-nitrogen and urea were about 508 (402-636), 10.2 (5.8-16.4) and 13.8 (10.4-18.4) mg per 100 ml of rumen liquor respectively (Ghosa1 *et al.*, 198l). Urea degradation rate in the rumen decreases, whereas plasma urea content increases with the corresponding increase in crude protein intaka (Emmanual *et al.*, 1976). Similar effect has been observed in the Bactrian camels. Type of feeding and time of sampling significantly influence the changes in ruminal nitrogenous constituents and increase in total nitrogen content in rumen is observed after 4-6 hours of feeding in the bactrian camels (Izmailov *et al.*, 1986) In the camelids end, some other ruminants greater proportion of the glomerular filtered urea is absorbed and recycled on the feeding of low protein diet (Schmidt-Nie1sen *et al.*, 1958, Engelhardt, 1978). Urea metabolism in camelids is close1y 1inked with the energy content of the diet (Engelhardt and Rubseman, 1979) and in water deprived camels the utilization of energy is also improved to certain extent (Farida *et al.*, 1979).

The metabolism of VFA in the camelids is somewhat different than the sheep end cattle. Glucose generation in true ruminants is about 50-75 mg %, whereas in the camels it is higher than 100 mg % and similar to monogastric animals (Yagil end. Berlyne, 1977, Chandrasena *et al.*, 1979, Kouider and Kolb, 1982.

Higher bicarbonate content in the rumen of camelids is said to enhance the absorption of VFA from the forestomach which is 2-3 times higher in llama in comparison to sheep goats (Rubsamen and Engelhardt, 1979). Larger amount of sodium and bicarbonates are present in the contents of the digestive tract of camels . The colon has very high water absorption capacity (Maloiy and Clamens, 1980). Metabolism of ketone is much lower in camels than the true ruminants because its main precursor butyrate is less efficiently metabolized die to low concentration of the enzymes 3-hydroxybutyrate dehydrogenase in the liver of camel than the sheep and goats. Oxidation of butyrate is very little in the herat and lungs of the camel (Emmanuel, 1980). The fatty acid profile of body fat of the camels is different from the true ruminants and hump fat contains more saturated fatty acids.

Rumen microbiology

Like true ruminants, the rumino-reticulum (C1 and C2) of the camelids is also inhabited by bacteria, protozoa and other micro-organisms responsible for the digestion and utilization of fibrous feeds and, non-protein nitrogenous substances for the supply of the nutritional requirements of the host animal. The population of bacteria has been found to be 7.18-26.20 (16.6 X 104) and ciliate protozoa 8.8-40.0 (19.1 X 10) per ml rumen liquor of Indian dromedary (Ghosal *et al.*, 1981). The population of protozoa in the rumen liquor of guanaco has been found to be much less than the goats (Harmayer and Hill, 1964). Ruminal protozoal population is less affected by water deprivation in camels than in sheep (Farid *et al.*, 1979). However, it is considerably influenced by the nature of diets and hour of sampling after the feeding of camels. Maxium number of protozoa has been counted 6 hours after the feeding in Indian dromedary (Table 16). Effect of diets on the proportion of different species has been found to be little (Bhatia *et al.*, 1986).

Table 16. Effect of diets on the rumen protozoa population.

Hours after	Diet A		Diet B	
Feeding	SRL	USRL	SRL	USRL
0	10.73 ± 0.89	15.13 ± 1.08	9.09 ± 0.38	13.93 ± 1.55
3	9.39 ± 0.62	14.13 ± 0.86	8.50 ± 1.18	12.44 ± 1.57
6	13.27 ± 0.14	19.93 ± 1.06	12.53 ± 1.63	18.09 ± 1.11
Mean	11.01 ± 0.60	16.42 ± 1.02	9.71 ± 0.67	15.85 ± 0.76
Per cent composition				
Entodinium	75.25 ± 1.16	74.83 ± 2.23		
Diplodinium	16.91 ± 1.14	18.00 ± 1.17		
Epidinium	6.33 ± 0.52	5.00 ± 0.04		
Holotrichs	1.50 ± 0.31	2.33 ± 0.42		

NB: Diet A is moth fodder + 2.5 kg pellets & Diet B is only moth fodder ad libitum.

Protozoa number is N X 10^4 per ml strained rumen liquor (SRL) or unstrained rumen liquor (USRL).

Digestion of feeds and nutrients

Higher digestibility of feeds and nutrients has been observed in the camelids in comparison to true ruminants (Fernandez-baca, 1966, Anonymous, 1971, Hintz *et al.*, 1973) But, lower digestibility of dry matter and crude protein has been observed in dromedary in comparison to zebu cattle on ad libitum feeding of poor quality dub (Cynodon dactylon) hay containing 6-7 per cent crude protein on dry matter basis. This was attributed to higher flow rate of digesta and lower retention time in the camel (Maloiy, 1972).

The proximate composition and digestibility of various organic nutrients of a shrub zinzru (Crotolaria medicagnea) leaves show the nutritional potential (Table 17) of fodder as sole feed. Mean dry matter intake 8.54 + 0.17 kg per day and containing about 10.86 per cent D C P and 61.66 per cent T D N on dry matter basis is capable to support considerable production in addition to maintenance of the camels in arid climate during winter season (Bhagwat *et al.*, 1991).

Table 17. Proximate composition and digestibility coefficients of zinzru leaves in Indian camels.

Particulars	DM	CP	EE	CF	NFE	Ash
Proximate composition (%)		14.66	2.78	33.45	41.88	7.24
Dig. Coeff. (%)	64.84	74.15	63.48	46.07	75.06	
SE +	0.88	1.45	2.02	3.31	0.97	

A significant increase in the digestibility of DM and organic constituents of diets on replacement of Lucerne hay with barley grain (Table 18) is similar to observations in other animals. Incorporation of barley grain in the ration reduced eating time, frequency of jaw movement and drinking during the meal period. Average values of CP, DCP, TDN, DE and ME of Lucerne hay and barley (by difference) were 17.8 and 12.4 %; 11.8 and 8.1 %; 55.3 and 79.9 %; 10.2 and 14.8 Mj/kg; and 8.4 and 12.8 Mj/kg of feed respectively (Bhattacharya *et al.*, 1988). The intake and digestibility of nutrients also increases significantly in lactating camels in comparison to dry camels (Table 19). Mean DM intake 8.78 ± 0.16 kg in lactating Indian camels was about 43 per cent higher than 6.13 ± 0.61 kg daily intake in the dry camels due to which TDN intake per kg W 0.75 was 33.7 ± 0.5 g in the dry and 48.0 ± 1.66 g in the lactating camels.

Table 18. Chemical composition and digestibility of lucerne hay and barley grain in Arabian camels.

Feeds	DM	OM	CP	NDF	ADF	Cellulose	Lignin
Chemical composition on DM basis (%),							
Lucerne hay	91.7	89.5	17.8	46.9	35.8	27.9	10.9
Barley grain	91.3	97.4	12.4	27.0	7.2	6.2	1.9
Digestibility coefficient,							
Lucerne hay	56.5	61.5	66.2	45.5	44.9	55.5	
Lucerne hay + barley (1:1)	69.4	73.6	65.5	54.7	45.2	58.9	
Barley grain	82.3	85.7	64.8	64.2	45.5	62.2	

Table 19. Digestibility coefficient of feed and nutrients in camels.

Animals type	DM	OM	CP	EE	CF	NFE
Dry	59.30	66.31	54.61	13.86	47.72	75.07
+SE	3.48	2.87	3.88	7.35	4.47	4.02
Lactating	62.65	67.95	58.76	26.34	45.48	79.13
+SE	0.77	1.66	0.68	2.52	2.71	2.57

Mean digestibility coefficients of oat hay, totora (Scorpus sp.) and oat silage in alpaca were 77.5, 79.1 and 71.2, and the values obtained in sheep 49.7, 66.4 and 54.6 respectively for the corresponding order of feeds were much lower (Fernandez Baca, 1966). Similarly, a comparative study with ponies, sheep and llamoids (Table 20) shows clear superiority of digestion efticiency in llomoids on the feeding of same diets (Hintz *et al.*, 1973). Table 20. Comparison of digestibility of diets in ponies, sheep and llamoids (llama and guanco).

Feed components	Ponies	Sheep	Llamoids
Ad libitum feeding of Alfalfa hay			
D M dig. (%)	64.8 ± 1.7	63.8 ± 1.1	71.5 ± 1.7
C P dig. (%)	65.7 ± 3.1	69.7 ± 0.2	74.7 ± 2.7
NDF dig. (%)	60.1 ± 0.6	58.5 ± 1.1	69.4 ± 2.4
ADF dig. (%)	46.7 ± 1.3	50.5 ± 0.2	61.0 ± 4.0
Cellulose dig. (%)	51.2 ± 3.0	64.8 ± 4.1	77.6 ± 0.9
Pelleted diet of timothy hay (33), yellow maize (53), soyabean meal (11), molasses (2) and dicalcium phosphate (1) parts :			
D M dig. (%)	69.7 ± 0.9	71.3 ± 1.7	78.0 ± 1.1
C P dig. (%)	68.8 ± 1.4	63.1 ± 1.0	69.2 ± 2.4
NDF dig. (%)	45.4 ± 1.7	44.7 ± 1.3	58.6 ± 3.0
ADF dig. (%)	29.3 ± 2.3	34.0 ± 0.4	38.7 ± 4.5
Cellulose dig. (%)	34.5 ± 2.3	39.4 ± 1.4	47.2 ± 5.2

The composition of diets and nutrient contents in the diets have significant effect on the performance of growing camels. An average 615, 404 and 340 g daily gain in the body weight of growing male camels has been observed on the feeding of pelleted concentrate at the rate of 15 g per kg body weight alongwith ad libitum lucerne hay, rhodes grass hay and ammoniated wheat straw in group 1, 2 and 3 respectively. The concentrate pellet, lucerne hay rhodes grass hay and ammoniated straw contained about 18.7, 13.8, 7.2 and 7.7 per cent C P and 2.80, 2.39, 2.08 and 2.10 Mcal ME per kg dry matter, respectively (Alfuraiji *et al.,* 1994).

Rearing of camel calf on milk substitute feeding

Neonatal calves pf dromedary weaned at 30 days of age may be successfully reared on the pail feeding of a good quality milk substitute or milk replacer normally used for rearing the young ones of other ruminants.a milk substitute composed of milk products, fat, minerals and other ingrediets used for lamb rearing was found suitable for the feeding of camel calves. This milk substitutes contained about 24% crude protein including 19% casein, 22% including 1% free fatty acids, 0.01% cellulose, 6.8% total ash, 1% calcium.0.72 % phosphorus. It was fortified it 40,000 IU of vitamin A activity and 8000 IU of vitamin D3 per kilogramme of milk replacer. Its solubility (misibility) was about

90% in warm water at 40°C. The milk substitute is reconstituted to contain about 15% of powder and fed at the rate of 1 litre per feeding thrice daily from 31-40 days, twice daily during 41-50 days and once daily during 51-60 day a alongwith ad libitum concentrate mixture containing 18% crude protein and lucerne hay. The feeding of concentrate mixture and lucerne hay continued upto 6 months of age. Average daily gain in body weight of calves during 30 days suckling was 700 g which decreased to 617 g during 60 days feeding of milk substitute and then to 560 g during 3-6 month of age, (Elias *et al.,* 1986).

Dietary energy concentration plays significant role in body growth of early weaned camel calves (Degan *et al.,* 1987). About 870 g daily gain in body weight of dromedary calves during 30 days suckling on whole milk on whole milk feeding indicates great potential of camel veal production. Average 32.5 kg body weight at birth increased to 58.5 kg at 30 days of age. Average milk intake has been found to be 12 to 18 per cent of body weight at different stages during 30 days of age i.e. 4, 6.6, 8 and 8.6 litres daily during 1-5, 6-15, 16-25 and 26-30 days of age, respectively. Camel calves learn to drink milk from pail or basin in about 5 days. Milk consumption per kg gain in body weight is about 8 litres. After 30 days of age, milk feeding is gradually reduced and the calves are offered good quality starter diet of about 18 per cent crude protein content alongwith legume hay (lucerne hay) which provided about 700 g daily gain in body weight from 31 to 60 days of age. Average body weight gain further decreased to about 550 g per day during 2-6 month of age, when milk was completely removed from the diet of the calves (Elias *et al.,* 1986). Similar potential of veal production in Arabian dromedary has been also observed (Degan *et al.,* 1987).

The birth weight of alpaca and llama cries is almost doubled in about two months of suckling. Suckling duration has been reported to range from 124 to 160 (average 140 ± 2.3) days in alpacas but in many cases it may continue upto next lambing. Weaning has adverse effect on the growth of cria for a short period of 7-8 days and thereafter gradually improves. The cries of advanced age spent little time on suckling (10.57 ± 1.10 minutes for 5.6 ± 0.58 sucks daily) and longer period for grazing (Pollard *et al.,* 1993).

References

Acland, P.B.E. 1932. Notes on the camel in eastern Sudan. Sudan Notes Rec., 15: 119.

Alfuraiji, M.M., Basmail, S.M. and Gamil, M.H. 1994. A note on relationship of plasma thyroxine and tri-iodothyronine rate to body weight in growing male camels. Anim. Prod., 59: 460.

Anonymous, 1971. Report of Veterinary institute for tropics and hight altitude ros., Lima, Peru.

Anonymous, 1992-93. Annual report of National Research Centre on camel. ICAR, Bikaner, India.

Asad, T. 1970. The Kababish Arabs: Power, authority and consent in a nomadic tribe, 263 pp. C. Hurst and Co., London.

Bhagwat, S.R. Pande, M.B. and Radadia, N.S. 1991. Nutritive value of zinzru (Crotolaria medicagneat beamlam) leaves for camels. Indian J. Anim. Nutr., 8: 311.

Bhatia, J.S., Ghosal, A.K. and Gupta, H.K. 1988. Rate of passage of digesta through the digestive tract of camel. Intern. J. Anim. Sci., 3: 45.

Bhatia, J.S. Ghosal, A.K., Gupta, A.K., Sharma, A.K. and Shekhawat, V.S. 1986a. Studies on unilaternal parotid secretion in camel (Camelus dromedaries). Indian Vet. J., 63: 18.

Bhatia, J.S., Ghosal, A.K., Raisinghani, P.M. and Tanwar, R.K. 1986b. Studies on rumen protozoa of camel (Camelus dromedaries). Indian Vet. J., 63: 109.

Bhatia, J.S., Ghosal, A.K., Sharma, K.E. and Shekhawat, V.S. 1984. Volume of rumen contents of camel. Indian vet. J., 61: 432.

Bhattacharya, A.N., Al-Mutairi, S., Hashimi, A. and Economides, S. 1988. Energy and protein utilization of lucerne hay and barley grain by yearling camel calves. Anim. Prod., 47: 481.

Bulliet, R.W. 1975. The camel and the wheel. 328 pp. Harvard Uni. Press, Cambridge.

Chandrasane, L.G., Emmanuel, B. and Gilanpour, H. 1979. A comparative study of glucose metabolism between the camel (Camelus dromedaries) and the sheep (Ovis aries). Comp. Biochem. Physiol., 62A: 827.

Church, D.C. 1988. The ruminant animal digestive physiology and nutrition. Prentice Hall, New Jersey 07632.

Cole, D.P. 1975. Nomads of the nomads. The Al-Murrah Bedouin of the Empty Quarter. 179 pp. Aldine, Chicago.

Cummings, J.F., Munnall, J.F., Vallenas, A. 1972. The mucigenous glandular mucosa in the complex stomach of two New World camelids, the llama and guanaco. J. Morphol., 137: 71.

Degan, A.A., Elias, E. and Kam, M. 1988. A preliminary report on the energy intake and growth rate of early weaned camel (Camelus dromadarius) calves. Anim. Prod., 45: 301.

Dellmann, H.D., Blin, P.C. and Fahmy, M.F.A. 1968. On the micro-scopic anatomy of the digestive tract in the camel. Revue Elec. Med. Vet. Pays Trop., 21: 1.

Dougbag, A.S.A.M. and Berg, R. 1981. Histological and histochemical studies on the pyloric mucosa of the camel's stomach (Camelus dromedaries). Anatomia Histologia embryologia, 10: 187.

Droandi, I. 1936. II cammello: Stora naturale, anatomia, fisiologia, zootecnica, patologia. 856 pp. Istituto Agricolo Coloniale Italiano, Florence.

Ehrlein, H.J. and Engelhardt, W. von. 1971. Untersuchungen uber die Magenmotorik beim Lama. Zentbl. Vet. Med., 8: 181.

Elias, E., Chohen, D. and Steimets, E. 1986. A preliminary note on the use of milk substitutes in the early weaning of Dromedary camels. Comp. Biochem. Physiol., 85: 117.

Emmanuel, B. 1980. Oxidation of butyrate to ketone bodies and CO_2 in the rumen epithelium, liver, kidney, heart and lung of camel (Camelus dromedaries), sheet (Ovis aries) and goat (Capra hircus). Comp. Biochem. Physiol., 65B: 699.

Emmanuel, B., Howard, B.R. and Emady, M. 1976. Urea degradation in the camel. Canaddian J. Anim. Sci., 56: 595.

Engelhardt, W. von. 1978. Adaptation to low protein diets in some mammals. Proc. Zodiac Symp. Adapt. Centre Agric. Pub. Document, Wageningen.

Engelhardt, W. von and Rubsamen, K. 1979. Review of the digestive physiology in camelids. IFS Intern. Symp. Camels, Sudan.

Farid, M.F.A., Shawket, S.M. and Abdel-Rahman, M.H.A. 1979. Observations on the nutrition of camels and sheep under stress. Proc. IFS Intern. Symp. camels, Sudan.

Fernandez-Baca, S. 1961-62. Rev. Fac. Med. Vet., Uni. San Marcos, Lima, Peru.

Fernandez-Baca, S. 1966. Utilization comparative de los forrajes por la alpaca yal ovino. Memorias V Congress Pana de Med. Vet. Y Zootecnia, 1: 352.

Field, C.R. 1979. Camel growth and milk production in Marsabit District, Northern Kenya. Proc. IFS Workshop on camels, Khartoum.

Gautheir-Pilters, H. and Dagg, A.I. 1981. The camel. Its evolution, ecology, behaviour and relationship to man. The University of Chicago Press, Chicago.

Gautheir-Pilters, H. 1972. Water intake of the dromedary in summery in the region of Beni-Abbes (North-west Sahara). Bull de I'Institut foudam D'Afrique, Noire, A. 34: 219.

Ghosal, A.K., Tanwar, R.K. and Dwarkanath, 1981. Note on rumen micro-organisms and fermentation pattern in camel. Indian J. Anim. Sci., 51: 1011.

Hansen, A. and Schmidt-Nialsen, K. 1957. On the stomach of camel with special reference to the structure of its mucus membrane. Acta Anatomiea, 31: 353.

Harmeyer, J. and Hill, H. 1964. The volume of protozoa in the rumen contents of goat and guanaco. Zntl. Vet. Med., 11A: 493.

Haller, R., Cercasov, V. and Engelhardt, W.V. 1986a. Retention of fluid and particles in the digestive tract of the llama (Lama guancoe f. glama). Com. Biochem. Physiol., 83A: 687.

Haller, R., Lechner, M. and Engelhardt, W.V. 1986b. Forestomach motility in the camel (Camelus dromedaries). Comp. Biochem. Physiol., 84A: 285.

Hintz, H.F., Schryver, H.F. and halberd, N. 1973. A note on the comparison of digestion by new world camels, sheet and ponies. Anim. Prod., 16: 303.

Hoppe, P., Kay. R.N.B. and Maloiy, G.M.O. 1974. Salivary secretion in the camel. J Physiol., 224-32.

Hoppe, P., Kay, R.N.B. and Maloiy, G.M.O. 1976. The rumen as reservoir during dehydration and rehydration in camel. J. Physiol., 254: 76.

Izmailov, T.U., Bagailov, E.B. and Mutaliv, A. 1986. Changes in nitrogenous substances in rumen contents of camel. Trudy Inst. Fiziol. A N Karakh SSR, 29: 124.

Jakhomola, R.C. 1992-93. In the annual report of the National Res. Centre on camels, Bikaner, India.

Kouider, S.A. and Kolb, E. 1982. Concentration of glucose and urea in serum of camel. Monatshefte fur Vet. med., 37: 140.

Leese, A.S. 1927. A treatise on the one-humped camel in health and disease. 382 pp. Haynes and Sons, Stanford Lines.

Leonard, A.G. 1891. The camel. Longman Green and Co., London.

Luciano, L. and Engelhardt, W. von. 1980. The fine structure of the stomach mucosa of the llama (Lama guanacos). 2. Cell Tissue Rec., 208: 519.

Maoiy, C.M.O. 1972. Comparative studies on digestion and fermentation rate in the forestomach of the one-humped camel and the zebu steer. Res. Vet. Sci., 13: 476.

Maloiy, C.M.O. and Clemens, E.T. 1980. Colonic absorption and secretion of electrolytes as seen in five species of East African herbivoroms mammals. Comp. Biochem. Physiol. 667A: 21.

Macfarlane, W.V. 1964. Terrestrial animals in dry heat: ungulates. In Handbook Physiology by Dill. American Physiological Society, Washington.

Mohammed, A.A. 1979. Histological and histochemical studies of the gastric mucosa of the third compartment of the camel, (Camelus dromedaries). J. Egyptian Vet. Med. Assoc., 39: 29.

Moir, R.J. 1968. Ruminant digestion and evolution. In: Handbook of Physiology. American Physiological Soc., Washington.

Mostafa, M.S., Aly, M.A., Ammar, S. and Aly, A.E. 1983a. Topography, morphology and duct system of the pancreas of the camel (Camelus dromedaries) Assiut Vet. Med. J., 10(20): 9.

Mostafa, M.S., Aly, A.E., Ammar, S. and Aly, M.A. 1983b. Blood vessels and nerves of pancreas of the camel (Camelus dromedaries). Assiut Vet. Med. J., 10(20): 15.

Mura, U., Mohamed, A.S., Osman, A.M. and Ipata, P.L. 1983. Comparison of amylases in blood serum and organs of the dromedary. Bollettino Sci. D., Somalia, 4: 29.

Ortiz, C., Cavero, J., Sillau, E. and Chueva, S. 1974. The parotid saliva of the alpaca (Lama pacos). Res. Vet. Sci., 16: 54.

Perrault, U. 1966. Description anatomique de deux chameaux. Mem. Acad. Sci., 1666.

Pilliet, A. 1885. Structure de la portion gaufree de l'estomac du chameau. Bull. Soc. Zool., France, 10: 40.

Pollard. J.C., Littlejohn, R.P. and Davis, G.H. 1993. Changes in live weight and behaviour of alpace dams and offspring following weaning. New Zealand Vet. J., 41: 161.

Purohit, M.S. and Rathor, S.S. 1962. Stomach of the camel in relation to that of the ox. Indian vet. J., 39: 604.

Qayyum, M.A. Fatami, J.A. and Mohajir, A.M. 1988. Scanning electron microscopic study of the lingual papillae of the one-humped camel, Camelus dromedaries. J. Anatomy, 160: 21.

Rubsamen, K. and Engelhardt, W. von. 1978. Bicarbonate secretion and solute absorption in forestomach of the llama. American J. Physiol., 235: 1.

Rubsamen, K. and Engelhardt, W. von. 1979. Morphological and function peculiarities of the llama forestomach. Anna. Res. Vet., 10: 473.

Schmidt-Nielsen, K. 1964. Desert animals: physiological problems of heat and water. Clarendon Press, London.

Schmidt-Nielsen, K., Crawford, E.C., Newsome, A.E. and Rawson, K.S. 1963. The metabolic rate of camels. Fed, Proc., 22: 176.

Vallenas, A. 1965. Some physiological aspects of digestion in the alpaca (Lama pacos). In: Physiology of digestion in the ruminants by R.W. Dougherty *et al.*, Butterworth, Washington.

Vallenas, A., Cumming, J.F. and Munnel, J.F. 1971. A gross study of the compartmentalized stomach of the two new world camelids, the llama and guanaco. J. Morph., 134: 399.

Vallenas, A. and Stevends, C.E. 1971. Motility of the llama and guanaco stomach. American J. Physiol., 220: 275.

Vorano, A.E. and Bertoni, J.A. 1984. biological and production parameters in the llama (Lama glama. Cuvier) on natural pastures of the high Andean plateau, with supplementation and different stocking rates. Rev. Argentina Prod. Anim., 4: 325.

Williamson, G. and Payne, W.J.A. 1978. An introduction to animal husbandry in the tropics. 3rd ed. Longman, Singapore.

Wilson, R.T. 1978, Studies on the livestock of souther Darfur, Sudan. V. Notes on camels. Trop. Anim. IIlth. Prod., 10: 19.

Yagil, R. and Berlyne, G.M. 1977. Glucose handling and dehydration in the camel. J. Appl. Physiol., 421: 680.

Yagil. R. and Etzion, Z. 1980a. Milk yields of camels (Camelus dromedaries) in drought area. Comp. Biochem. Physiol., 67A: 207.

Yagil, R. and Etzion, Z. 1980b. the effect of drought conditions on the quality of camel's milk. J. Dairy Res., 47: 159.

Yagil, R., Etzion, Z. and Ganani, J. 1978. Camel thyroid metabolism: effect of season and dehydration. J. Appl. Physiol., 45: 540.

❑❑❑

Chapter 4

Reproduction and Breeding

Male Reproductive System

The stud male camel is one of the most important animal in the herd. A breeding male can sire 20 to more than 50 females in a season. In pastoral herds, little attention is given for the selection of camel bulls in most of the cases but in some countries even the herders use some selection traits like high growth rate, milk production and wool production. In case of riding camels, the race performance and indurance are the main critaria of selection. In general, most of the breeding males are selected on the basis of vigour, size, conformation and the production performances of their parents (Hartley, 1979). Replacement males are usually selected at 3-4.5 years of age in case of bactrian and dromedary camels (Terentjev, 1951, Matharu, 1966) and at 1.5-2 years of age in cameloids (Fernandez Baca, 1975).

Anatomy of the Male Reproductive Tract

The reproductive tract of male camel is formed of the main organs and the accessory organs or glands. The main organs include a pair of testes contained in a pouch of skin called scrotum. The testes are continued into the duct system made of the epididymis, vas deferens, urethra and penis. The accessory glands present in the camselids are the prostate and bulbourethral or Cowper's glands. The seminal vesicles are not present in the camels (Tayeb 1948, Mobarak *et al.*, 1972).

The scrotum

The visible part of a male reproductive organs is the scrotum situated protruding in the perineal region as in the dogs. It a skin sac tightly encapsulating the testes and closely attached to the body. The oval shape scrotum appears clearly divided into two parts by a median band (raphe). Few small heirs are present scattered on the scrotum. The scrotum is normally covered with the tail but it is seen in the standing animals. The left part of the scrotum is a little larger than the right part due to corresponding difference in the size of testes. The size of scrotum is larger during the rutting season due to increase in the size of more active testes (El-Wishy and Omar, 1975).

The testes

The oval shaped testes are presented horizontally in the perineal region. The left testis is little 1arger than the right one. The posterior border of the testis is free and convex and ahterior border is almost straight except some depression along the attachment of the epididymis on the anterior-dorsal aspect. On attaining puberty at about 3 years of age, the length is 7-10 cm and weight is 80-110 g (Tayeb, 1951-52, El-Wishy and Omar, 1975). In older camels of 6-10 years or age the average length, breadth and thickness of the testes are 9.07, 5.08 and 4.43 cm respectively, and weight is about 92 g (El-Wishy and Omar, 1975). The testes of camels contain less number of cells per gramme of tissue, when compared with the testes of bulls, buffaloes, rams and boars (Osman and El-Azab, 1974). The testes protrude during the rutting season due to enlargement caused by increased development of the interstitial cells but dehydration for longer period for 3 weeks or more has adverse effect. The weight of testes in adult camels is generally more than 165 g and may be upto 253 g in some large size males during the rut. The weight is less than 140 g during the quiscent period (Charnot, 1963a,b).

The intratesticular excurrent ducts or seminiferous tubules can be differentiated into four parts, viz, the tubuli seminiferi ,contorti, the terminal segment of the seminiferous tubules, the tubuli recti and the rate testis. Each tubulus restus is further delineated into the receptacle, narrow main part and wider distal part. The seminiferous tubules taper progressively alongwith which the germ layers are gradually lost until the epithelium becomes columnar with a few spermatozoa. The columnar cells of the terminal part are considered to be the modified Sertoli cells (Osman, 1986). The diameter of seminiferous tubules is larger in the rutting season and these contain 5-6 layers of germ cells in various stages of differentiation and abundant mitoses. The degeneration of germ cells begins with the end of rutting season when degeneration of spermatozoa occurs. The tubules become gradually devoid of spermatozoa and vacuolation becomes consipicuous. In the non-rutting season, the degeneration is well advanced, spermatozoa and mitoses are almost absent and diameter of the tubules is greatly reduced. Again regenerative changes begins with the start of the breeding season concurrent with the disappearance of the degenerated cells due to phagocitosis by the Sertoli cells (Charnot, 1964, Novo, 1970, Abdel-Raouf *et al.,* 1975). High levels of 17- Keto-steroids is observed in the urine of rutting males (Charnot, 1958). The neuro-secretary cell of the anterior pituitary gland are more active during rut (Santini, 1964). The alpha LH and the beta FSH secreting cells of the anterior pituitary gland are hyperactive in the rutting males and least active during the sexual rest (Charnot and Racadot, 1963). Blood testosterone rises from 1.5-3 ng per ml during sexual rest to about 36 ng per ml in rut. The concentration is similar in the smelly brown secretion of the neck glands (Yagil and Etzion, 1979).

The reproductive activity in males is not completely stopped in the non-rutting season but the rate of spermatogenesis is highly decreased (Abdel-Raouf *et al.,* 1975). Some changes of reproductive activity have been seen in the testicular inter-stitial cells even during the non-rutting season (Tingari *et al.,* 1979) and frequency of the seminiferous epithelium cycle is significantly not influenced by seasonal changes (Osman *et al.,* 1979).

The epididymis

The epididymis is formed of caput (head), corpus (body) and cauda (tail). The caput epididymis is a flat structure, the corpus epididymis is narrow and continues with the third part, the cauda epididymis (Tingari and Moniem, 1979, Osman and Ploen, 1986). The tail of the epididymis is very closely associated with the testicular surface by an epididymal ligament (Leese, 1927). The ductus epididymis is lined by pseudostratified ciliated columnar epithelium containing mainly two types of cells, viz, the tall columnar cells and the basal cells (Goswami *et al.,* 1994). The height of epididymal epithelium is males dehydrated for three weeks (Charnot, 1963a).

Histological structure and histochemistry of the epididymis of dromedary males have been studied in detail (Tingari and Moniem, 1979, Singh and Bhardwaj, 1980, Goswami *et al.,* 1994). The duct of the initial segment of epididymis presents a regular and smooth contour. The lumen is wider (about 200 µm) and contains fewer spermatozoa. A typical pseudostratified ciliated columnar cells of about 130 µm average height are situated on a distinct basal membrane form the epithelial lining. The oval nuclei may show mitotic activity and the supranuclear cytoplasm in these cells is vacuolated and eosinophilic. Average height of the stereocilia is about 23 μm (Tingari and Moniem,1979). The histological structures of the initial, middle and terminal parts of the corpus and cauda epididymis of the Indian camels revealed considerable regional variation is size of different components (Table 21). The elongated, spherical and dense nuclei in parts other than the initial caput are present mostly in the central part of the cells. The height of the epithelial cells and microvilli reduces progressively towards the cauda epididymis but diameter of the tubules and their lumen increases (Tingari and Moniem, 1979, Singh and Bhardwaj, 1980, Goswami *et al.*, 1994).

Table 21. Mean size (μm) of different structures of the epididymis.

Structures	Caput epididymis			Corpus epididymis		Cauda epididymis	
	Initial	Middle	Terminal	Initial	Terminal	Initial	Terminal
Diameter of tubules	285	350	275	275	340	612	625
Diameter of tubular lumen	165	190	100	100	245	475	516
Height of epithelium	38	65	35	40	25	30	25
Height of stereocilia	10	15	15	10	7	3	3
Size of nucleus	7	9	7	7	5	5	5
Thickness of tunica muscularis	16	15	25	18	18	25	40

The vas deferens or ductus deferens

The vas deferens of camel is highly convoluted, straightening only towards the distal part. The spermatic cord is thickened and fairly long and contains the vas deferens, pampiniform plexus, spermatic artery, nerves, lymphatic vessels and internal cremester muscle. The lumen of vas deferens is formed of longitudinally folded mucosa. The internal inguinal ring is very narrow (Leese, 1927). The ductus deferens of alpaca has a muscular layer divided into two strata against three strata of muscular layer in other animals (Osorio and San Martin, 1966). The lumen of ductus deferens in scrotal region is formed of longitudinal mucosal folds and frequently contains masses of sperms. It is lined with pseudostratified columnar cells studded with stereocilia. The later are shorter than that in the ductus epididymis and the sperm heads are found attached with the stereocilia. Cytoplasm of the cells is acidophilic and foamy except in the supranuclear zone, where it appears homogeneously granular. The nuclei are oval and situated in the basal part of the epithelium and their chromatin is coarse and dispersed near the periphery. Another kind of cells in the epithelium are the basal cells which are generally oval to spherical and vacuolated. The lamina propria-submucosa is thin and made of circularly arranged collagen and reticular fibres but devoid of elastic fibres. The nuclei of varying size and capillaries are present in the fibrous mess. The tunica muscularis is formed of an inner thick layer of circular muscle and outer thin 1ayer or longitudinal muscle fibre bundles. The tunica serosa is made of closely knotted collagenous and reticular fibres (Degen and Lee, 1982, Goswami *et al.,* 1994).

The ampulla ductus deferentis contains larger number of glands embedded in the entire lamina propria-submucosa. The epithelium of the initial part of the ampulla is formed of pseudostratified non-ciliated columnar to cuboidal cells with vesicular nuclei containing uniformly dispersed chromatin in the basal part of the cells. The shape of nuclei is elongated oval to spherical. The luminal border and subapical cytoplasm of the epithelial cells is deeply eosinophilic and vacuolated in the remaining part of the supranuclear cytoplasm. The secretary character of the cells is shown by Bleb like protrusions from the apical border. The epithelial lining in middle and terminal segments of ampulla ductus deferentis is formed of simple columnar to simple cuboidal cells. The mucosal folds gradually reduces and the epithelial layer is almost flat in the terminal segment (Ali *et al.,* 1978, Degan and Lee, 1982, Goswami *et al.,* 1994).

The penis

The penis of camel is long and firm cylindrical organ contained in a massive and triangular conical sheath or prepuce. The sheath hangs from the abdomen in the inguinal region like a mammary gland. The penile prepuce is darker in colour with few small hairs scattered on the surface and posteriorally directed orifice. The muscles of the prepuce are arranged in three groups i.e., an anterior, a posterior and the lateral. The anterior muscles are largest and the lateral ones are the weakest. Contractions and relaxations of these muscles control the movements of the penis and also the constriction and dilatation of the preputial orifice. All three groups of muscles insert into the inner surface of the skin enveloping the free preputial part of the penis (Tayeb, 1948, Mobarak *et al.,* 1972). Whole of the preputial part is covered with keratinized stratified squamous epithelium devoid of any glands or hair.

The average length of penis of the dromedary is about 58 cm (Leese, 1927, Nagpal *et al.*, 1987) but great variation ranging from 37.5 to 50 cm in some breeds of Indian camels (Khan and Kohli, 1973) and 57.6 to 67.5 cm in Egyptian camels (Mobarak *et al.*, 1972) has been reported in different studies. The penis can be delineated into three segments, viz. radix (root), corpus (body) and pars libra penis (free part of penis). A prescrotal sigmoid flexure is formed by the middle part of the penis and the length of penis may also be distinguished as pre-sigmoid, intra-sigmoid and post-sigmoid of about 17.5, 25 and 17.5 cm and comprising about 29, 42 and 29 per cent of the total length respectively (Tayeb, 1948). The diameter of the penis gradually decreases from the root towards the free preputial part (Nagpal *et al.*, 1987). Average diameter of the root, middle part and free terminal part of the penis is about 2.23, 1.64 and 0.42 cm respectively (Mobarak *et al.*, 1972). The cranial end of the free preputial part is twisted and directed dorsally and a little towards left forming a hook-shaped curved terminal process of about 2.2 cm length. It is hard to feel due to the presence of a ring of hyaline cartilage (Nagpal *et al.*, 1987). The preputial orifice is directed posteriorally in elevated position for providing protection to the genital organs from the hot sand in squating posture. This also causes backward direction of the urine which is splashed with the tail on the posterior part of the body for evaporative cooling.

The penis originates in the region of the ischiotic arch and its root is formed of three cavernous bodies. Two corpora cavernosa penis are situated dorsally and a single corpus spongiosum ventrally in the midline. The last one contains urethra. The cavernous bodies are covered by a thick tunica albuginea made of outer longitudinal and inner circular layers of collagenous fibres bundles. Some elastic fibres are also present in the collagenous fibre bundles but these are abundant in the tunica albuginea, covering the corpus spongiosum (Nagpal *et al.*, 1987). Some oblique collagen fibres are also present with the circular layer of the tunica albuginea (Degan and Lee, 1982). Rows of chondrocytes are found in inner fibrous layer of the tunica albuginea. The chondrocytes are also present in the cavernous tissue in the root and body of the penis in the areas adjoining the tunica albuginea. The number and dispersal area of chondrocytes vary greatly between the individuals. The corpus cavernous penis changes into a ring of hyaline cartilage containing many blood vessels in its core in the region of the curved terminal process. The cartileginous ring is surrounded by many caverns and elastic fibres (Mobarak *et al.*, 1972, Degen and Lee, 1982, Nagpal *et al.*, 1987).

The corpus spongiosum contains larger cavernous space in the corpus cavernous penis and the number of theses spaces decreases from the root of the penis to the area of the sigmoid flexure and then again increases largely towards the preputial region. The inter-cavernous tissue is similar to the corpus cavernous penis but contains more elastic fibres. The wall of the blood caverns contains several longitudinally oriented smooth muscle fibre bundles projecting into the lumen (Nagpal *et al.*, 1987).

The urethra

The urethra is a muscular duct receiving semen from the ampulla ductis deferentis and secretions from the accessary sex glands. It is centrally located in a groove covered with corpus spongiosum in the thick layer of tunica albuginen. Dorsally at the base of the terminal process a 0.46 to 0.5 cm long pointed processus urethrae is present (Mobarak *et al.*, 1972, Nagpal *et al.*, 1987). In this region, the corpus spongiosum is transformed into a bar of hyaline cartilage (Degen and Lee, 1982, Nagpal *et al.*, 1987). The urethra is lined with the layer of transitional epithelium except in the region of urethral process, which is lined by keratinized stratified squamous epithelium. The lamina propria-submucosa is formed of dense fibroelastic tissue surrounded by many venules and veins providing it the appearance of cavernous tissues. The urethra is covered with the fibroelastic tissue seperating it from the corpus spongiosum. On its ventral aspect, a consipicuous thickening of fibroelastic tissue forms a longitudinal ligament like structure which continues through out the length of penis except the processus urethrae. The urethra is well protected dorsally as well as ventrally from the pressure of the engorged cavernous tissue. The subepithelial tissue is highly vascular and contains many encapsulated nerve endings. The lymphocytes are also seen aggregated at many places (Nagpal *et al.*, 1987).

The accessory sex glands

In camelids, only two accessory sex glands are found along the penis. These are the prostate and bulbo-urethral or Cowper's glands. The seminal vesicles present in other ruminant species are absent in the camelids. The discoid prostate gland is formed of two lobes (pars prostata) connected with an isthmus. The prostate gland is situated on the dorsal aspect of the pelvic urethra. The colour of prostate gland iş dark yellow and size is 3-7 x 5 cm. The isthmus is a thin band. Several ducts from the prostate gland drains into the urethra. The whitish almond shaped bulbo-urethral or Cowper's glands are two in number measuring 2.5 x 1.2 cm. These glands are situated on either side of the terminal part of the pelvic urethra (Leese, 1927, Tayeb, 1948).

Protrusion of penis

The penis does not protrude out of the prepuce due to penopreputial adhesions in the young age. The shedding of adhesions occurs with the increase in age and it is probably dependent on the production of androgens. The shedding of penopreputial adhesions is completed during the progressive maturity and animals become capable of copulation. The protrusion of erected penis out of prepuce occurs at 3-4 years of age in the camels and 1.5–2 years of age in the cameloids (Sumar and Garcia, 1986).

Spermatogenesis

The spermatozoa are formed from the germinal cells of the seminiferous tubules. The epithelial lining of the seminiferous tubules contains two types of basic cells, the germ cells and the Sertoli cells. The germ cells divide and grow continuously from the from the periphery towards the lumen. The development process of the germ cells begin with the formation of spermatogonia which progressively develop into spermatocytes, then spherical spermatids and finally elongated spermatids. The stern cells are called spermatogonia, which are divided several times before the formation of spermatocytes. The spermatogenic cycle of the seminiferous epithelium in camels has been delineated into eight stages of about 21.83, 11.07, 13.42, 8.24, 10.32, 9.35, 9.25 and 16.43 per cent frequency in the progressive stages (Osman *et al.*,1979). The eight stages of the cycles of the seminiferous tubules (Osman and Ploen, 1986) may be briefly described as follows:

Stage 1 : At this stage only one generation of round spermatids are formed.

Stage 2 : Elongation of the nuclei of spermatids starts and their staining reaction increases.

Stage 3 : The spermatids are grouped in bundles and elongated nuclei are dark stained.

Stage 4 : The spermatocytes are present in meiotic division alongwith few young spermatids and also the bundles of older elongated spermatids.

Stage 5 : At this stage, two generations of spermatids are found simultaneously. The older spermatids have elongated nuclei and the youngers are spherical spermatids. Innermost layer of the seminiferous tubules is formed by the elongated spermatids.

Stage 6 : The round spermatids are present towards the lumen of the tubules and the elongated spermatids are deeply embedded in the cytoplasm of the Sertoli cells.

Stage 7 : At this stage bundles of elongated spermatids are found at different levels in the epithelium.

Stage 8 : The elongated spermatids line the lumen of seminiferous tubules, whereas a few free spermatozoa are present in the lumen.

The Spermatogonia

The spermatogonia are present in the basal lamina and classified on the basis of the length of the area of contact with the basal lamina and also the size and shape of the cell and nucleus, and the number of chromatin encrustations in the nucleus as follows :

i) Typical spermatogonia type A
ii) Typical spermatogonia type B, and
iii) Intermediate type of spermatogonia.

i) **The spermatogonia type A :** These are flattened large cells with broad area of contact with the basal membrane and remaining surface is covered by adjacent Sertoli cells. The nucleus is mostly oval with long axis parallel to the basal lamina. The chromosome is homogeneous and finely granular with some marginal heterochromatin material. Sometimes, a large nucleus situated centrally or accentrally may be present. The density of cytoplasm is variable. The other organelles found in the spermatogonium are mitochondria, ribosomes and polyribosomes. The mitochondria accumulate at one side of the nucleus. The Golgi apparatus is less clear and endoplasmic reticulum is scarce.

ii) **The spermatogonia type B :** These are round in shape having variable but smaller area of contact with the basal lamina. The nucleus is spherical and possesses more peripheral chromatin than in type A cells. The chromatin is less uniform and areas of more condensed chromatin are found in between light areas. One or two nuclei are seen either associated with the nuclear envelope or free in the karyoplasms or chromosome. Cytoplasm contains grouped mitochondria and many free ribosomes and polyribosomes.

iii) **Intermediate type of spermatogonia :** These are highly variable cells intermediate in characters between type A and B.

Primary spermatocytes

In the process of development these cells are present in the following five stages :

i) Leptotone stage : At this stage, the cells are detached from the basal lamina and present completely covered by the cytoplasmic processes from the adjacent Sertoli The cell and nucleus are rounded nucleolus is distinct. The cytoplasm contains some endoplasmic reticulum but the mitochondria did not yet have dilated cristae.

ii) Zygotone stage : More cisternae of endoplasmic reticulum is formed with a few attached ribosomes. Grouping of mitochondria and dilatation of cristae begin. The nucleolus is often seen in the nucleus and synaptonemal compeses appear between the pairs of the chromosomes.

iii) Pachytene stage : This stage is comparatively longer and could be observed alongwith many other stages of development of the seminiferous epithelial cycles. The mitochondria are grouped containing dense inter-mitochondrial substance possessing dilated cristae. Well formed Golgi appartus is present. The formation of proacrosomal vesicles containing granules begins. The quantity of endoplasmic reticulum in the form of long parallel cisternae is increased enormously which is distributed throughout the cytoplasm but more accumulation towards the periphery of the cell. Marginal heterochromatin is conspicuous and synaptonemal complexes are common.

iv) Late pachytene-diplotene stage : The cell is now large with prominebt Golgi apparatus possessing pro-acrosome vesicles with granules. Long cisternae of endoplasmic reticulum are prominent but synaptonemal complexes are not observed.

v) Cells in final stage of meiosis : It is rather difficult to distinguish morphologically the first and second meiotic divisions. At this stage, the mitochondria are distributed throughout the cell. The chromatin material is present in typical arrangement of the different phases of cell division. Secondary Spermatocytes, the cells and their nuclei are smaller. The nucleus is more homogeneous. Inter-mitochondrial substance is present free in the cytoplasm and endoplasmic reticulum is plenty.

Spermatids

The spermiogenesis is a continuous process and it may be divided into several phases or stages. Seasonal reduction in consonence with the breeding season occurs in spermatogenesis in the camels but aspermiogenic condition does not arise in otherwise normal males (Abdel-Raouf *et al.*, 1975, El-Wishy and Omar, 1975). Various stages of spermiogenesis (Osman and Ploen, 1986) are as follows :

1. Golgi phase : The cell and nucleus are round add the later contains some marginal heterochromatin and a nucleolus. The Golgi apparatus becomes prominent and its vicinity many small and large size vesicles are found. These vesicles collected to form the large acrosome vesicle containing electron dense acrosome granules which approach the nucleus and form a small depression and then start to spread over the nuclear surface. The chromatid body and the tail aula are situated near the Golgi apparatus and an invagination of the plasma membrane appears around the tail aula. Close to the nuclear envelope or in the vicinity of the Golgi apparatus electron dense material of the cytoplasm bound by cisternae of the endoplasmic reticulum is present. The mitochondria possessing dilated cisternae are randomly dispersed throughout the cell.

2. Cap phase : The cell and nucleus still remain round and the later contains a homogeneous chromatin pattern with marginal heterochromatin. About one-third circumference of the nucleus is covered by the achrosome containing dense granules. Many long cisternae of endoplasmic reticulum are present. A deep implantation fossa is formed end implantation of the tail takes place during late cap phase. At this stage, longitudinal columns start start to develop forming the annulus.

3. Early acrosome phase : The nucleus is placed accentrical in the cell and the acrosome is directed towards the basal lamina. Both cell and nucleus begin to elongate. The nucleus contains homogeneous pattern of chromatin and few patches of heterochromatin. The zone of heterochromatin is very narrow and it is continuous under the acrosome but disintegrated in the post-acrosomal area of the nucleus. Almost half of the circumference of the nucleus is enveloped by the acrosome and anterior projection of acrosome granules begins. A perinuclear ring is formed due to accumulation of the dense material on the plasma membrane at the posterior margin of the acrosome. The post-nuclear region contains Golgi apparatus, whereas the tail region contains the dense rounded structure surrounded by membranes and the chromatoid body. Now the implantation fossa and structure of the future neck piece is formed.
4. Mid acrosome phase : The nucleus becomes more elongated with coarser chromatin threads in comparison to previous phase. The anterior end of the nucleus tapered and the acrosome granule is further elongated anteriorly. The nuclear cover is elevated from the chromatin material in the post-acrosomal region of the nucleus.
5. Late acrosome phase : The condensation of chromatin threads is more pronounced, further elongation of nucleus takes place and nuclear cover is more elevated than the previous phase. The condensation of chromatin is uniform throughout the nucleus. The density of acrosome granule and remaining portion of the acrosome is same. The perinuclear ring starts to migrate towards the posterior nuclear pole. The centriolar adjunct is clear, manchette is well formed and dense material forming the collar of annulus is formed.
6. Transition between the late acrosome and maturation phases: Anterior elongation of the acrosome becomes very long and asymmetrical. The entire acrosome is filled with dense material. The perinuclear ring is pushed posteriorly which subsequently disappears alongwith the microtubules of the manchette. Now the nucleus is very dense and homogeneous. There is complete formation of post-acrosomal sheath and the posterior nuclear pockets alongwith the structures of neck region of tail. The appearance of spindle shaped body is not clear and only a few helically arranged microtubules are present. The migration of

annulus towards the anterior pole of the future principal piece begins.

7. Maturation phase : In this phase, a short bulbus body is formed due to retraction of the asymmetrical anterior elongation of the acrosome forming its equatorial segment. Arrangement of the mitochondria begins around the developing mid piece of the tail for the formation of mitochondrial sheath. There is complete formation of connecting piece, the axoneme, the outer dense fibres and fibrous sheath of the tail. Most of the cytoplasm of the maturing cell is demarked just before the spermiation which is left as residual class in the epithelium at spermiation. The intercellular bridges left between the groups of residual bodies are phagocytosed by the Sertoli cells.

Factors affecting the characteristics of testes

The development of testes and their physiological functions are influenced by several factors like age, genetic factors and various environmental factors like plane of nutrition, supply drinking water, climatic changes and vigour of the male. Hormones play significant role in regulating the functions of the testes. Dromedary and bactrian camels attain puberty at about 3 years of age and sexually mature at 6-10 years of age (El-Wishy and Omar, 1975, Chen and Yuan, 1980). In alpaca, the lumen in the seminiferous tubules appears before 12 months of age and spermatozoa as well as Leydig cells are present at 15-18 months of age (Montalvo *et al.,* 1979). The level of plasma testosterone at 11 months old alpaca is similar to that in adults (Losmo and Coyotupa, 1979). The testes remain functional throughout the year but activity is more during the rutting season (Abdel-Raouf *et al.,* 1975). Extended dehydration had adverse effect on spermatogenic activity (Charnot, 1963). Effects of age and season on some characteristics of testes (Table 22) have been studied in detail in dromedary males (Abdel-Raouf *et al.,* 1975).

Characteristics of Semen

The semen is light grey to milky white and viscous at the time of collection. After 10-15 minutes of keeping at room temperature, its viscosity decreases significantly becoming reasonably fluid and sperms become motile. The common characteristics of semen of different species have been compiled (Table 22). All the characteristics of dromedary semen except the volume have been found to be similar on collection by two methods (Musa *et al.,* 1993).

Table 22. Characteristics of semen

Species	Ejaculate volume, ml	pH	Sperm count nX $10^6/mm^3$	Live sperm %	Normal sperm %	Motility %	Mass motility	Source
Dromedary	8.5 (4.3-12.6)	8.6	0.4	55	-	-	-	Abdel-Raouf and El-Naggar, 1978
do	5.0 (1.0-9.0)	7.8 (7.6-8)	0.8 (0.4-1.3)	43 (25-66)	84 (60-92)	-	1.8 (1.0-2.6)	Tingari *et al.*, 1986
do (by AV)	7.5	7.4	0.33	82	64	50.5	-	Musa *et al.*, 1993
do (electro-ej.)	3.9	7.4	0.33	81	65	49.7	-	do
Bactrian	7.72 ± 2.28	-	0.62 (0.22-1.25)	-	95 (93-98)	-	-	Chen and Yuan, 1980
Alpaca	12.5	-	0.6	-	-	-	-	Sumar and Garcia, 1986

Spermatozoa

As usual the spermatozoa are formed of an elliptical or paddle shaped head, a short mid piece and a long tail. The shape of sperm is similar to ram's sperm (Leese, 1927) but size is shorter than the sperm of bulls and buffaloes (Abdel-Raouf and El-Naggar, 1965). Some information available on the measurements of dromedary sperms have been summarised (Table 23).

Table 23. Measurements (µm) of spermatozoa of dromedary.

Measurement of sperm	1	2	3	4
Length of head	5.35	5.6	5.5	5.5 ± 0.4
Width of head	3.42	-	2.5	3.6 ± 0.5
Length of acrosome	-	2.4	-	2.2 ± 0.1
Length of mid piece	7.38	7.3	7.0	6.9 ± 1.0
Length of tail	35.60	34.2	35.0	35.6 ± 1.7
Total length	48.38	47.2	50.0	48.0 ± 1.0

NB: 1- Khan and Kohli, 1973; 2- Andel-Raouf and El-Naggar, 1978; 3- Osman and Ploen, I986 and 4- Tingari et al., I986.

Some biochemical constituents of the secretion of accessory sex glands, ampulla and urethra.

In a sporadic study, wide variations have been observed in the concentrations of fructose and citric acid in the secretion of prostate gland, Cowper's gland, ampulla and urethra (Table 24). In addition to this constituents the content of protein and lipids has also been reported in the seminal plasma of dromedary (Table 25). However, these observations were limited to 3-8 animals only (El-Manna *et al.*, 1986).

Table 24. Fructose and citric acid content in sex glands secretions.

Secretion	Fructose (mg/dl)		Citric acid (mg/dl)	
	Range	Mean	Range	Mean
Prostate gland				
(a) Pars disseminate	5.0-23.8	9.8 ± 0.7	8.5-18.5	15.8 ± 1.8
(b) Corpus prostatae	8.8-50.9	21.6 ± 1.4	19.8-63.5	35.3 ± 2.2
Cowper's gland	17.0-96.3	34.0 ± 2.1	21.5-44.5	36.0 ± 3.1
Ampulla	23.8-131.2	41.2 ± 2.5	4.5-50.1	24.9 ± 1.9
Urethra	5.6-25.5	10.7 ± 0.8	0.0-18.5	7.2 ± 0.9

Table 25. Biochemical constituents of seminal plasma in different individual of dromedary.

Constituents		Camel 1	Camel 2	Camel 3	Camel 4
Fructose (mg/dl)	Range	17.0-32.0	17.0-40.0	15.0-31.0	14.0-25.0
	Mean	24.2 ± 3.2	27.0 ± 5.6	22.3 ± 1.4	20.3 ± 2.1
Citric acid (mg/dl)	Range	5.0-12.0	10.0-30.0	5.0-13.0	5.0-10.0
	Mean	7.2 ± 1.2	14.1 ± 1.6	10.8 ± 1.4	7.0 ± 0.9
Protein (mg/dl)		790 ± 10	780 ± 6	780 ± 6	750 ± 8
Lipids (mg/dl)		98 ± 12	68 ± 3	135 ± 10	48 ± 5

The Female Reproductive System

The anatomy of the female reproductive organs of the camel resembles more to the mare's genital organs than the ruminants genitalia. A pair of ovaries and the tubular genital organs form the main reproductive system. The tubular organs include a pair of short oviducts or fallopian tubes, a pair of uterine herms, a small and muscular corpus uteri or body of the uterus, a compact cervix, long vagina, vestibule, hymen and the vulva. The internal genital organs are supported by the bread ligament attached dorsally on either side of the sublumbar region and laternal aspect of the pelvic wall. The bread ligament is normally demarcated into mesovarium, mesosalpinx and mesometrium supporting the ovaries, oviducts and uterus respectively. The weight of the whole genial organs ranges from 194 to 376 g in the camels (Shalash, 1965) but it is much less in the cameloids. The mammary glands are considered as the accessory sex organ because its development, functions and utility are closely related with the reproductive functions in the females. The reproductive organs are formed in the embryonic stage and had slow growth during the prepubertal life but there is sudden increase in the growth with the onset of the puberty (Table 26). The increase in the tubular parts is many folds (Pareek *et al.*, 1981)

Table 26. Average measurements of the genital organs of the Indian dromedary female.

Measurement of the organs (cm)	Age of the female		
	3 days	1 month	Adult
Right ovary attached to free border	1.4	1.7	3.0
Right ovary from anterior to posterior border	0.7	1.6	4.5
Left ovary attached to free border	1.1	1.7	3.5

Left ovary from anterior to posterior border	0.8	1.2	3.5
Length of the right uterine horn	3.4	1.2	3.5
Length of the left uterine horn	4.2	5.0	15.4
Length of the corpus uteri	0.5	0.8	8.0
Length of the cervix	3.2	4.7	7.6
Length of the vagina	7.6	11.2	34.8
The vulva	Small	moderate	large

The ovaries

The ovaries are two in number, the right ovary and the left ovary and are present in the abdominal cavity supported by the mesovarium. The ovaries are fully developed but small and smooth without any follicular activity at birth and in early post-natal life. Average size of the left ovary at birth is about 1.1 cm X 0.8 cm and that of right ovary is about1.4 cm X 0.7 cm which increases to about 1.7 cm X 1.2 cm and 1.7 cm X 1.6 cm at one month of age and about 3.0 cm X 3.5 cm and 3.0 cm X 4.5 cm respectively in the adult Indian camels (Pareek *et al.*, 1981). There is great variations in the dimension of ovaries (Table 27) which is mainly due to follicular activity in the adult female (Table 28). The anoestrus ovary is normally oval and thin. In the mature animals, the surface of the ovaries is pear shaped and uneven due to the formation of many ovisacs on its surface (Shalash, 1965, Arthur *et al.*, 1985).

Table 27. Average size of ovaries in camels.

Observation	Size of ovaries (cm)	Weight (g)	Source
1	-	3.66 - 8.51 ± 1.49 ± 2.66	Shalash, 1965
2	3-6 X 2.5 – 4	-	Abde *et al.*, 1968
3	3.3 X 2.0 X 1.3	10	Chahrasbi *et al.*,
4	4.0 X 2.5 X 0.5	-	Arthur *et al.*, 1985

Tab1e 28. Mean diameter and weight of ovaries during different reproductive stages (Shalash, 1965).

Ovaries	Anoestrus		With Graffian Follicles		Without Corpora lutea of preg.	
	Right	Left	Right	Left	Right	Left
Diameter (cm)	1.82 ± 0.35	1.90 ± 0.32	2.09 ± 0.35	2.15 ± 0.36	2.28 ± 0.28	2.33 ± 0.33
Weight (g)	3.66 ± 1.49	3.89 ± 1.63	5.51 ± 2.69	5.47 ± 2.62	7.94 ± 2.50	8.51 ± 2.66

In the pregnant camels, the shape and size of the ovaries change with the progress in gestation (Table 29) and the ovary possessing an active corpus luteum. The difference in weight is mainly due to the weight of the corpus luteum of pregnancy (El-Wishy *et al.*, 1981).

Table 29. Effect of the stage of gestation and the size of corpus luteum on the weight of the ovary.

Days of pregnancy	Weight of the ovary (g)		Size of Corpus luteum	
	With CL	Without CL	Diameter (cm)	Weight (g)
60	11.00	4.67	2.25	6.73
120	9.00	3.00	2.00	4.00
180	9.08	3.67	2.20	5.25
210	8.75	2.75	2.15	5.25
240	11.19	4.92	2.15	4.88
270	9.02	4.21	2.26	5.19
345	10.05	4.30	2.15	4.90
390	8.00	2.50	2.30	5.00

The oviducts

Each oviduct is about 22 to 28 cm long and tortuous tubular structure suspended in the mesosalpinx part of the broad ligament. The oviduct may be delineated into four parts, the finger shaped fimbriae, the funnel shaped infundibulum, the ampulla and the isthmus. The fimbriae are situated in the bursa near the ovary. The lumen of the ampulla is 4-4 mm in diameter at its ovarian opening in the depth of the fimbriae. The isthmus is narrower and less coiled and its diameter is 1-2 mm. It opens into the uterine cornu through a narrow orifice at the top of a papilla of 3-4 mm height (Tayeb, 1953, Arthur *et al.*, 1985).

The uterus

The uterus of the camels is as usual bicernual and large. Its larger portion is situated in the abdominal cavity and some part in the palvic cavity. The uterus alongwith the cornua are is found hanging in the mesometrium part of the broad 1igament. The dorsal aspect of the uterus is convex, smooth, reddish white and less dense in texture while the lower aspect is flat. The corpus uteri is short and thick. There seems to be minor effect of follicular activity on the size of the uterus including the horns (Table 30). A slight increase in the length of corpus uteri may be observed (Shalash, 1965). The length of corpus uteri of the Indian camels is about 8 cm which is quite high (Pareek *et al.*, 1981). It appears that some part of apparently conjoined horns was also measured as corpus uteri.

Table 30. Effect of ovarian activity on the size of uterus.

The uterus	With follicular growth	During anoestrus
Corpus uteri		
Length (cm)	2.11 ± 0.29	1.85 ± 0.40
Diameter (cm)	5.39 ± 0.90	5.84 ± 0.94
Right horn of uterus-		
Length (cm)	13.42 ± 1.76	13.37 ± 2.15
Diameter (cm)	3.73 ± 0.63	3.73 ± 0.69
apex	2.35 ± 0.41	2.44 ± 0.44
Left horn of uterus-		
Length (cm)	17.45 ± 2.86	17.53 ± 3.29
Diameter (cm)	4.29 ± 0.90	4.99 ± 0.91
apex	2.87 ± 1.67	3.07 ± 0.69

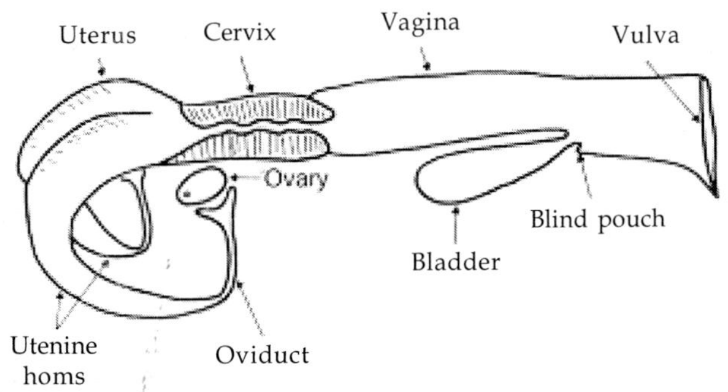

Fig. 3 : Schematic diagram of female reproductive system of camel

The cornua uteri are closely associated for some distance from the corpus uteri and anterierly separated in the T-shape which is different from the Y-shape in cows. The left horn is invariably larger than the right horn (Shalash and Nawito, 1964, Joshi *et al.*, 1978) and such is the situation even at birth and in early life (Pareek *et al.*, 1981). The mucous surface of the uterus including the horns is smooth and devoid of the cotyledons (Lesbre, 1903, Tayeb, 1951, Shalash and Nawito, 1964).

The cervix

The cervix or neck of the uterus is a short and muscular passage joining the uterus with the vagina. The cervical passage is plugged during the pregnancy. The length of cervix in Indian camels ranges from 3.5 to 7.6 cm and diameter is about 5.5 cm (Joshi *et al.*, 1978, Pareek *et al.*, 1981). There is also difference in size due to follicular activity. Average length 5.32 ± 0.98 cm and diameter 5.96 ± 0.92 cm of the cervix during follicular activity were more than the corresponding 4.96 ± 1.25 cm and 5.79 ± 0.99 cm during the non-functional or anoestrus ovaries (Shalash, 1965). The cervix contains 3-4 rows of mucosal folds or ridges and their size changes with the ovarian activity. The cervix protrudes about 1 cm into the vagina terming two, a dorsal and a ventral blind sac. The mucosa of the cervical canal forms longitudinal folds and terminates as a prominent crest terming the internal os uteri (Shalash, 1965, Joshi *et al.*, 1978).

The vagina

The light pink colour vagina is about 35 cm long in the Bikaneri females (Joshi *et al.*, 1978, Pareek *et al.*, 1981). It is an elastic tubular organ containing both longitudinal and circular mucosal folds in the vaginal walls and contain the canals of Gartner and the glands of Bartholini in the vaginal walls originating in the region of the external cervical opening (Tayeb, 1953).

The vestibule

It is a short ridge at the opening of the urethra. A hymen is present at the vestibule and persistent hymen is also a cause of for about 0.12 per cent of the total incidences of infertility in the camels (Shalash, 1965, Joshi *et al.*, 1978).

The vulva

The external female genital part is vulva. Average size is 6.26+0.02 cm long and slightly increases to 6.52+0.78 cm during estrus (Joshi *et al.*, 1978).

Ovulation

The release of ovum from the mature Graafian follicle is known as ovulation. In almost all camelids except some sporadic incidence in alpaca, ovu1tion is not spontaneous but induced by semen deposition in vagina either by coitus or by artificial insemination (Barmintsev, 1951, Shalash, 1965, England *et al.*, 1971, Musa and Abusineina, 1976, Chen and Yuan, 1980). In the bactrian camel, ovulation occurs after 30-48 hours of coitus. Ovu1ation can not be induced by mechanical stimulation of the cervix. If two follicles mature together, both ovulate in response to copulation. However, ovulation does not occur even on copulation at the time of the start of regression of the follicles (Chen *et al.*, 1980). Both ovaries are found active during the breeding season and multiple ovulation occurs in more than 10 per cent females but multiple birth is rare (San Martin, 1961, Shalash, 1965). Post-coital ovulation interval is about 26 hours in the cameloids (Fernandez Baca,1993). Some factor present in seminal plasma is responsible for ovulation because it could not be induced by insemination of washed camel sperms. The nature of ovulation inducing factor in the seminal plasma is not known but it is rapidly absorbed from the vaginal and uterine walls and respond quickly as in one study, one of the four naturally mated female bactrian camels ovulated inspite of washing their vagina after 10 minutes of copulation (Chen *et al.*, 1985).

A follicular wave covers the period of time between the acceptance of the male by the female. This is accompanied with changes in the ovaries. Re-acceptance of male by the same female is an indicator for the start of a new follicular wave of about six days duration. The follicular wave may be divided into four stages, viz. mature follicular stahe, atretic follicular stage, non-follicular stage and growing follicular stage. Copulation or deposition of semen or seminal plasma (Table 32) is essential for ovulation (Nawito *et al.*, 1967, Chen and Yuan, 1980).

Although in all camelids ovulation is induced by copulation or deposition of semen in the vagina, some unusual factors have been observed to induce ovulation in aplacas and one of the 20 females ovulated only by the sight of a male (Table 32) but coitus and administration of ovulatory hormones are affective for larger higher ovulation (Fernandez Baca *et al.*, 1970, Chen *et al.*, 1985).

Tab1e 31. Factors affecting ovulation in bactrian and alpaca females.

Factors affecting ovulation	Females used	Females ovulated	Per cent ovulation
Bactrian females			
Natural service	25	25	100
Insemination with fresh live semen	12	11	92
Insemination with frozen (-10°C)			
Semen containing dead sperms	10	9	90
Insemination with seminal plasma	8	6	75
Insemination with accessory sex glans			
secretion without sperms	4	4	100
Coitus with vasectomised camel	3	3	100
Flushing of vagina 10 minutes post-coitus	4	1	25
Insemination with washed camel sperms	7	0	0
Insemination with bull semen	7	5	71
Insemination with buck (goat) semen	5	0	0
Insemination with boar semen	5	0	0
Insemination with skim milk	7	0	0
Injection of hormone (1000-1500 IU, HCG)	4	4	100
Alpaca females			
Sight of the male	20	1	5
A single non-ocoital mount by malc	13	2	15
Mounting + artificial insemination	9	3	33
Interrupted service	10	6	60
Sterile service	22	17	77
Sterile service + AI	21	18	86
Single service by stud male	44	36	82
Multiple service	10	7	70
Injection of hormone (750 IU, HCG)	28	28	100

All camelids are seasonal breeder except near the equator where seasonal variation is very little. The seasonality of breeding influences ovulation (Table 32) and calving rate in different monthe (Table 33). During breeding season females have more large follicles in comparison to non-breeding season. In alpacas, ovarian follicles take 3-5 days for maturing to ovulatory size (Bravo and Sumar, 1989).

Table 32. Monthly distribution of ovulation and fertility in alpaca.

Month	Females No.	Mated %	Females No.	Ovulated %	Fertilization %
May	10	10.64	8	80	63
June	12	12.77	8	67	88
July	9	9.57	8	89	67
August	15	15.96	9	60	89
September	15	15.96	10	67	83
October	13	13.83	9	69	88
November	10	10.64	9	90	100
December	10	10.64	9	90	67

Sources : Fernandez Baca *et al.*, 1972.

Table 33. Calving rate during different months in dromedary.

Month	Herd 1		Herd 2		Herd 3	
	No.	%	No.	%	No.	%
January	60	9.43	25	13.97	331	33.50
February	40	6.29	12	6.70	289	29.25
March	30	4.72	10	5.59	152	15.38
April	42	6.60	12	6.70	50	5.06
May	80	12.58	30	16.76	13	1.32
June	60	9.43	22	12.29	1	0.10
July	58	9.12	14	7.82	-	-
August	42	6.60	11	6.15	-	-
September	50	7.86	18	10.06	-	-
October	42	6.60	10	5.59	3	0.30
November	60	9.43	12	6.70	9	0.91
December	72	11.32	3	1.68	140	14.17

Sources: Herds 1 & 2, Wilson, 1986; Herd 3, Khanna *et al.*, 1990.

Age at first service

The age at first service under pastoral management is more or less the cyclic period just after the onset of puberty. It is generlly longer due to inadequate feed supply in the arid zones of the tropical and subtemperate climatic areas. Under suck conditions of hot or cold desert, the age at first service ranges from 3 to 5 years (Mares, 1954, Chen and Yuan, 1984, Chowdhury, 1986, Khanna *et al.*, 1990, Abdel-

Rahim *et al.*, 1994, Chapman, 1985). The age at first service can be reduced to 2-3 years by better feeding and management (Arthur *et al.*, 1985, Abdel-Rahim *et al.*, 1994, Kamoun *et al.*, 1994). Vicuma and llama species are bred at about one year of age (Dennier De Latour, 1954, Fernandez Baca, 1975).

The oestrus or heat

The physiological changes in the reproductive organs of the females for the manifestation of receptivity for mating is known as oestrus or heat.

The signs of oestrus

The characteristic changes in the behaviour of the breedable females preparing for mating are manifested by several sequential and characteristic signs. The appearance of such signs is seasonal in the dromedaries under most of the agro-climatic conditions. The camel owners are generally familiar with the common signs of oestrus accordingly they arrange the breeding of their in heat, whereas in mixed herds on pastures the females in oestrus themselves find their mate. There is large variation in the oestrus behaviours of the camels and the cameleids.

A female camel in oestrus likes the company of males until mating takes place and the mating continues in breeding season until the receptive female conceives. A female camel in heat strongly rejects her seperation from the male and often sits down, when forcibly driven away for working or riding (Singh and Prakash, 1964, Joshi *et al.*, 1978). During first one or two days, the females in oestrus become off feed, restless, run with raised tail frequently moving up and down or carried on a side, push the males and bleats continuously. The vulva is swollen and there may be some discharge from the vagina (Singh, 1966). A strong foul odour is emitted from the vulva of the females in heat which can be smelt over long distance. This has an exciting effect on the male camels and attracts them. The vulva lips are swollen and contracts frequently. The cervix is relaxed and moist and 1-3 fingers could easily to the cervix (Shalash, 1965, Joshi *et al.*, 1978). The behaviour is often unpredictable and erratic and suck females are excited even when pack loads are put on their flanks. Frequent micturitien in small quantity is observed during the first half of the oestrus duration (Droandi, 1915, Yasin and Wahid, 1957, Joshi *et al.*, 1978).

The vagina is edematous, moist and pinkish in colour during the pre-oestrus period. The females allow the male to sniff their genitalia by raising tail but do not permit coitus and run away, when forced for assuming mating position. During oestrus, the vagina is still moist and becomes red due to engorgement of the blood vessels and remains so upto the middle of the oestrus period and thereafter its colour gradually faints turning red to pink during the later half of the oestrus period and becomes pale after the end of oestrus. The vestibular is also red to pink during the oestrus find also moist. The vaginal mucous membrane appears sticky and discharge is not observed after the mid oestrus and moistness gradually subsides towards the end of the oestrus. The vaginal swears contains flat cells with characteristic cosinophilic cytoplasm and pyknotic or faint streak like nuclei. Transitional cells and least mature cells with folded edges are also identified alongwith a few basal or parabasal cells. The uterine cornua are turgid at the beginning of the oestrus which gradually subsides after middle of the oestrus. On the fourth day, slight flaccidity is observed in both the horns. The left horn is normally larger than the right one and also more turgid during the oestrus. Several Graffian follicles without any corpus luteum of pregnancy are present on both the ovaries and appear like small vesicle mostly over the dorsal and ventral borders (Joshi *et al.*, 1978, Musa, 1979).

During parading of a male teaser the female in oestrus is attracted and approaches the teaser. She sniffs his genitalia, prepuce and perineal region. She comes close to the male, bites the face, muzzle and ears of the male and twists her neck around the neck of the teaser. Now both partners come to proximity of each other and remain for some time in head to head position This is quickly followed by adoption of a sitting posture for copulation and the female in oestrus remains sitting for some time even after the male is removed temporarily. When mounted by the male, she expresses her desire to be mated by extending her neck upwards and backwards closer to the face of the mounted male. Another female in heat also comes near the copulating male and often bites his ear, remains near him and watch the coitus eagerly (Joshi *et al.*, 1978). The other camels in the herd are aterted at this time and encircle around the copulating camel (Arther *et al.*, 1985). If a female does not conceive, she again comes in heat after 10-13 days of anoestrus period (Novea, 1970, Joshi *et al.*, 1978).The signs oestrus in different llama species are somewhat different than the camels. The alpaca female in heat immediately assumes the mating posture when approached by the male. A female in oestrus comes near the mating female and watches copulation. Some females in oestrus may also mount other female (Fernandez Baca *et al.*, 1970). The oestrus is almost continuous with irregular and sporadic period of dioestrus in the female llamas. A continuous uninterupted oestrus period of 30 days duration has bean reported in many females and in some, it may extend upto 50 to 90 days. The females respond very quickly when approached by the male and acquire mating posture. A courting period longer than 4 minutes frequently terminates without mating or an aggressive male resorts to force mating (England *et al.*, 1971). The non-oestrus females of alpaca and llama strongly reject the male by running away, kicking and spitting on the dale (Fernandez Baca *et al.*, 1970, England *et al.*, 1971).

The oestrus period or oestrus duration

The duration of oestrus in the bactrian and dromedary camels is normally 4-6 days (Gupta *et al.*, 1978, Joshi *et al.*, 1978 and Chen and Yuan, 1984). However, short oestrus period of one day duration and long oestrus period of 8-21 days duration may also occur (Barmincev, 1951, Parkes,1969, Williamson and Payne, 1978). About two months long duration of oestrus in dromedary - (Islamy, 1960) appears to be on wheresay basis.

In alpaca and other cameloids, the oestrus duration is highly variable and ranges from 4-35 days which again occurs for 4-30 days after a short non-receptive lapse of 1 or 2 days dioestrus in the virgins. In multiparous alpacas, it ranges from 7-36 days in the start of the breeding season and reoccurs in non-bred females after an usual short dioestrus interval of 1 or 2 days duration (San Martin, 1961). It is generally believed that the llama species remain in heat continuously in the breeding season until conceive or male refuses to mate (Guilbrige and Moro, 1965). Some information on oestrus period have been compiled (Table 34).

Table 34. Oestrus period in different camelids.

Species	Oestrus period (days)	Source
Bactrian	1-21	Barmincev, 1951
	4-6	Chea and Yuan, 1984
Dromedary	4-5	Gupta *et al.*, 1978
	4-6	Joshi *et al.*, 1978

	1-7	Parkes, 1969
Alpaca, virgin	4-35 (first)	San Martin, 1961
	4-30 (later)	
Parous	7-36 (first)	
	2-26 (later)	
	21-36	

The oestrus cycle

The dromedary camel is a seasonal breeder and breedable females show oestrus at intervals during the breeding season in most parts of the northern hemisphere (Hira, 1947, Novoa, 1970, Arthur *et al.*, 1985, Wilson, 1989). In the Indian camels, 4-5 oestrus cycles may be observed in the females which are not yet bred (Gupta *et al.*, 1978). In the breeding season, the females are receptive for 3-4 days at a tine. This is followed by 10-12 days of anoestrus period (Joshi *et al.*, 1978). The factors like rainfall nutrition and management way overside the effect of photoperiod and breeding may occur throuout the year near the equator but with variable intensity (Merkt *et al.*, 1990). A breeding periodicity occurs in the camels which is higher in the cold and rainy season (Bhargava *et al.*, 1965, Shalash, 1965, Khanna *et al.*, 1990). The domestic bactrian camels of the central Asian countries are generally polyoestrus and bred throughout the year while the wild or feral camels show seasonal oestrus cycles (Bosaev, 1938).

The camelids exhibit regular and predictable oestrus cycle. The oestrus behaviour is shown interrupted by irregular and sporadic periods of dioestrus (San Martin *et al.*, 1968, England *et al.*, 1971). Some times short dioestrus is overlooked and the alpaca females are considered to be in oestrus throughout the breeding season (Guilbridge and Maro, 1965). A break or non-receptive period of one or two days between the oestrus periods of 4-36 days (mostly 21-36 days) observed by San Martin *et al.* (1968) is much shorter than the average 38 to 70 days dioestrus, when females are not bred (England *et al.*, 1971). In alpaca appearance of oestrus has been normally observed after 13 days of the previous non-fertile mating (Fernandez Baca, 1975).

The pattern of sexual activities in the camelidae females is not yet fully known and needs detail observations. The length of oestrus cycles in different species has been compiled (Table 35).

Table 35. Oestrus cycle length in different species.

Species	Oestrus cycle (days)	Source
Bactrian	19 (14-24)	Chen and Yuan, 1984
Dromedary	23.4 (20-25)	Joshi *et al.*, 1978
	28	Musa and Abusimiena, 1978
	25-40	Yagil and Etzion, 1984
	24.2	Wilson, 1984
Llamas	Irregular and unpredictable cycles	San Martin *et al.*, 1968

Post-partum oestrus interval

The occurrence of post-partum. oestrus is highly variable. It is as short as one day after calving (Barmicev,1951) but generally 14-25 days after calving in the bactrian camels (Barmicev, 1951). The first oestrus after parturition in stall fed dramedaries has been found to be 25-40 days (Yagil and Etzion, 1984) and in Arabian camels it was still variable as evident from 29 post-partum interval (Abdel-Rahim *et al.*, 1994). Such short post-partum oestrus interval shows that sexual activities, specially the ovarian activity are little affected by suckling and lactation. Inspite of short post-partum interval, the females fail to conceive under most of the conditions in the same season and normally they are mated after several month of calving. However, on good feeding and management annual births has been common in some parts of Kenya (Yagil and Etzion, 1984).

Almost all cameloid species exhibit oestrus in 24-48 hours of parturition but with very little fellicular growth (Novea, 1970). The fellicle growth capable of ovulation in response to copulation. is normally observed from fourth day post- partum and maximum fertility occurs after 10 days of parturition (Sumer *et al.*, 1972). Annual birth is quite common in llamas and alpacas (San Martin, 1961).

Age at first conception

Average age of dromedary camels under pastoral management add under usual non-pastoral management ranges from 3 years to more than 5 years in dromedaries (Hira, 1947, Mares, 1954, Beniwal and Chowdhury, 1984, Chowdhury, 1986, Khanna *et al.*, 1990). However, there is enough scope of considerable reduction in the age at. first conception by improving the feeding end management in early life. It has been brought down to 28.7 and 31.8 months in the farm born and purchased yearling females dromedaries of Tunisia by feeding them at optimum level under standard management of an organised farm (Kamoun and Wilson, 1994). The age at first conception has been reduced to only about two years on good feeding and management in Saudi Arabia (Abdel-Rahim *et al.*, 1994) . Age at first conception in Indian camels is generally more than 1470 days which has been lowered to about 1245 days by better feeding and management (Beniwal and Chowdhury, 1984).

The bactrian camels are capable to conceive at 3-4 years of age but in practice first breeding is generally delayed by one or two years. The Astarkhari camels of steppes and its crossbreds with Kazkh are mostly bred at about 4 years of age (Terentjev, 1951) and in other areas after 4 years of age (Chen and Yuan, 1984, Chapman, 1985). Vicuna and llamas mostly conceive at about one year of age (Fernandez Baca, 1975).

Sexual activities in early life can be induced by the use of gonadotropin and other hormone preparations and the camels on good feeing may be bred successfully at less than two years of age (Yagil and Etzion, 1984).

Age at first calving

Age at first calving in most of the dromedaries is 3.5 to more than 5 years in the tropical countries (Hire, 1947, Mares, 1954, Matharu, 1966, Khanna *et al.*, 1990). It is 4-6 years in the bactrian camels (Terentjev, 1951, Chapman, 1985). However, camels have produced calves at about 3 years of age on feeding at high plane of nutrition and good management (Arthur *et al.*, 1971, Abdel-Rahim *et al.*, 1994). Fertile oestrus in well fed dromedary heifers of two years of age resulting into normal calving has been induced by the administration of follicle stimulating hormone for three consecutive says (Yagil and Etzion, 1984).

Number of service per conception

So far very little information on limited number of animals is available. The breedable females continue to copulate during the oestrus period until conceive or become anoestrus due to passing of time or infertile mating. About 4-5 oestrus cycles have been observed in the female camels during a breeding season in India (Gupta *et al.*,

1978). The number of service per conception normally ranges from 1 to 3 in the bactrian camels but a few females may not conceive even after several matings which has been reported to be due to the failure of ovulation in an otherwise normal female (Barmincev, 1951). Similar situation is encountered in dromedaries. An average 1.87, 1.75, 2.75, 2.12 and 2.71 services per conception has been observed on breeding the females on the first, second, third, fourth and fifth day of the oestrus period respectively and the number of service per conception increased on increasing the mating time after onset of the oestrus. Optimum time of breeding appears to be within 48 hours of the onset of oestrus (Gupta *et al.*, 1978). An average two service per conception may be required in the camels (Abdel-Rahim *et al.*, 1994).

Since llama, alpaca, guanico and vicuna leave in flocks and mating occurs several times during the season, it has not been feasible to determine the number or service per conception.

Gestation length / Pregnancy duration

The gestation length in the bactrian and dromedary camels is normally more than one year (Podberezkin, 1951, Mehta *et al.*, 1962, Chen *et al.*, 1980, Beniwal and Chowdhury, 1984, Chapman, 1985) whereas in small size species of South American cameloids, it is normally less than one year (Denneler De Latour, 1954, San Martin *et al.*, 1968, Strain and Strain, 1987). There is non-significant effect of the parity and age of the dam or sex of the calf in uterus on the gestation length but variation due to individual and location is quite high (Islamy, 1950, Yasin and Wahid, 1951, Mehta *et al.*, 1962, Chen *et al.*, 1980, Chowdhury, 1986, Khanna *et al.*, 1990).

The length of gestation in different species of the camels and cameloids is highly variable. Therefore, considerable number of observations made under different climatic and managemental conditions have been compiled (Table 36).

Table 36. Gestation length in different camelidae.

Species and factors	Gestation period (days)	Source
Dromedary camel	370	Iwema, 1960
Iran	365 (12 month)	Islamy, 1950
Israel, general	345-360	Yagil and Etzion,
stall fed	365-395	1984a, b
Pakistan	336-364	Yasin & Wahid, 1951

Old Russia	388	Blagovescenskii,
1963		
do	384	Dzhumagulov, 1979
do	13 month	Meredov, 1984
non-specified location	308-364	Leopard, 1894
do	336	Bodenheimer, 1954
do	370-375	Arthur *et al.*, 1971
India	398 + 2.1	Vyas, 1985
(a) Effect of parity		
First calving	389.9 + 2.1	Mehta *et al.*, 1962
Second onwards	390 + 2.4	
(b) Effect of calf sex		
Male calves 389.3 + 3.2		
Female calves	390.6 + 2.7	
Male calves 403.4 + 4.1	Shri Ram *et al.*, 1977	
Female calves	405.3 + 5.5	
Male calves 391.7 + 15.2	Chowdhury 1986	
Female calves	380.4 + 17.3	
Male calves 389.7	Khanna *et al.*, 1990	
Female calves	388.8	
Bactrian camel		
Kazakhastan	13-14 month	Podberezkin, 1951
Russia (old)	406	Blagovescenskii,
1963		
do	412	Dzhumagulov, 1979
do	406 or more	Dahl & Hjort, 1976
China	402 + 11.5(374-419)	Chen *et al.*, 1980
Bact. X Drom or		
Reciprocal hybrids 398	Dzhumagulov, 1979	
Alpaca, Huacaya type	342 (325-358)	San Martin *et al.*, 1968
Suri type	345 (326-361)	
Guanicoe & Llama	308	Cabrera & Yepes,
1940		
Vicuna	280	do

Calving interval or Inter calving period

Post partum oestrum may be shown one day after calving in camels (Barmicev, 1951) and 24-48 hours after parturition in llamoids

(Novoa, 1970). Fertile rating occurs after 14-25 days of calving in bactrian (Barmicev, 1951), 17-41 days in dromedary (Yagil and Etzion, 1984, Abdel-Rahim *et al.,* 1994) while maximum fertility in llamas and alpaca has been observed on breeding at 10 days post-partum (San Martin, 1961, Sumar *et al.,* 1972). However, larger number of bactrian and dromedary females are bred after 9-12 months of calving (Table 37) due to which calving interval is about 2 years in most of the dromedary and bactrian females (Hira, 1947 Islamy, 1950, Iwema, 1960, Podberezkin, 1951, Blagovenscenskii, 1963, Aueljbekov, 1967, Chapman, 1985). On good feeding and better management calving interval may be reduced to less than 18 months in bactrian (Terentjev, 1963) and 365-395 days in stall fed dromedary (Yagil and Etzion, 1984). Inter-calving period decreasses with the increase in parity but in aged females again increases (Khanna *et al.,* 1990).

Table 37. Effect of various factors on calving interval in camels.

Factor	Number	Calving interval	Source
Bactrian camel			
General feeding	-	2 years	Terentjev, 1963
Good feeding	-	1.5 years	do
Dromedary camel			
Stall fed	-	365-395 days	Yagil & Etzion, 1984
Effect of parity-			
(a) India, First	-	799 + 19 days	Khanna *et al.,* 1990
Second	-	784 + 16 days	
Third	-	741 + 12 days	
Fourth	-	741 + 19 days	
Fifth	-	709 + 16 days	
Sixth & more	-	872 + 59 days	
(b) Kenya, First	190	588 + 15 days	Wilson, 1986
Second	149	557 + 16 days	
Third	77	571 + 20 days	
4th-7th	44	565 + 26 days	
Effect of herd-			
Ngare Ndare	99	578 + 18 days	
Kisima	89		523 + 19 days
Galana	191	599 + 14 days	
01 Mairor	81	582 + 21 days	
Total	460	570 + 11 days	

Effect of calf sex-		
Female calves	218	574 + 15 days
Male calves	242	566 + 15 days
Effect of survival of calf-		
Abortions	69	541 + 23 days
Pre-weaning death	91	533 + 22 days
Post-weaning survival	300	636 + 15 days
Effect of calving month-		
January	39	570 + 33 days
February	17	583 + 47 days
March	25	579 + 38 days
April	37	529 + 31 days
May	58	548 + 26 days
June	40	599 + 32 days
July	47	543 + 31 days
August	27	624 + 42 days
September	41	567 + 32 days
October	27	577 + 37 days
November	46	594 + 30 days
December	56	528 + 28 days

Fertility rate and calving rate

The percentage of conception in a herd or flock is defined as the fertility rate and that of calving or lambing as the calving rate. Sometimes the two terms are intermingled which causes confusion. Calving rate or birth rate is generally lower than the conception rate. Such incidences are more common in different species of camelidae. The fertility and calving rates are influenced by several factors like the kind of feeding in stall fed animals, herbage cover and nutritional quality of vegetation available for browsing / grazing on pastures and range land, lactation length and milk yield, month of calving, body condition of the breedable females and number of breeding males, etc. Inspite of about 90.6 per cent conception rate in the camels (Kazakh and Asterkhan breeds) the calving rate has been only about 51.4 per cent which indicated considerable loss of embryos in bactrian camels (Terentjev, 1951). During the same period from other part of the central Asia, only 21.4 per cent conception rate has been reported and the cause of low fertility has been assigned to failure of follicle development. However, this information was recorded on a small herd of only 33 breedable bactrian females (Barmincev, 1951). Different records of calving rate show great variation ranging from 21.4 to 65 per cent, in the bactrian end 50 to 70 per cent in the dromedary herds (Table 38).

The calving rate in llamas is significantly influenced by the stocking rate on pastures besides other factors. High stocking rate of more than one animal per hectare on a pasture of about 983 kg annual dry matter production caused considerable loss of production and depletion of the herbage cover (Vorano and Bertoni, 1984). The fertility rate in alpaca and other species is significantly increased by the use of alternate breeding system. An increase in usual about 50 per cent calving rate to about 80 per cent calving in alpaca flocks bred by alternate mating system has been reported on good pastures (Novoa *et al.,* 1973).

Table 38. Birth rate in camelids.

Species, type etc.	Birth rate (%)	Source
Bactrian	21.4	Barmincev, 1951
(Kazakh & Asterkhan)	91.6 (Concep)	Terentjev, 1951
	51.4 (Birth)	
	46.7	do, 1963
	43	Yuzlikaev & Akhmediev, 1965
	65	Aueljbekov, 1967
	40	Keikin, 1976
Dromedary, Grabbra	34	Watsons, 1969
Somali	52.25	do
Bikaneri	69-85	Chowdhuri, 1986
India,		
Sudan, (Darfur)	70	Wilson, 1978
Llama species	50-60	Guilbridge & Moro, 1965
Llama, stocking rate-		
0.5 / ha	46.6	Vorano & Bertoni, 1984
1 / ha	20.0	
2 / ha	6.6	
Alpaca,		
normal management	50	Novoa *et al.*, 1973
alternate mating & better management	80 approx.	

Alternate mating system

The breeding season in llama species is usually extended from December to March which is rainy season in Peru, Bolivia, Chile and Argentina. During this period, high quality pasture grasses are abundantly available for the grazing. Thus, the animals maintain good condition. In alternate mating system, initially 10- 15 breedable females are left with a breeding male in several groups for 7 days. After this period, the males are removed to resting pens for 7 days and another set of unused males are left with the females in the same manner. After rest the previous males are again put to the groups of females but their previous groups are changed. This cycle of 7 days association followed by 7 days rest and then change of 'harm' or drove is repeated during the whole breeding season. The mating is very intense during the first two days and remains more or less so far 5 days, when males are first placed with the females, and an aggressive male can serve as many as 12 females on the first day of exposure. However, sexual activity diminishes at a fast rate during successive days and by seventh day the males are mostly reluctant to serve despite the availability of several receptive females in the drove (Fernandez Baca, 1975). Such effect of alternate mating on increased breeding has also been observed in the camels (Marie and Anouassi, 1986).

Site of Pregnancy

In camelids, both ovaries are active but left ovary is some what more active than the right one. Cross pregnancies are common feature in camelids due to high migration of ova to left horn. More than 95 per cent foetii develop in the left horn in the bactrian (Chen and Yuan, 1980), dromedary (Shalash, 1965) and New World cameloids (Fernandez Baca *et al.*, 1973).

Pseudopregnancy

Occurrence of pseudopregnancy is common in alpaca which is generally duo to high incidence of azoospermic males in the flock (San Martin, 1961). As high as one-third females in an alpaca flock may be found to show the signs of pseudopregnancy (San Martin *et al.*, 1968). In dromedary, presence of active corpus luteum in few females with patent cervix has been often considered pseudopregnancy (Shalash, 1965). Since ovulation is induced by coitus in camelids, the reason of pseudopregnancy appears to be mainly azoospería associated with high desire of bearing the foetus in such females.

Parturition

Conspicuous changes occur in the abdomen, mammary gland and external genitalia of the pregnant camels about 2-3 weeks prior to parturition. These signs intensify as the time of parturition approaches. On the appearance of these signs, the pregnant females are kept under close observation. The signs of approaching parturition or premonitory signs are characterized by upward cocking of the tail, distension of abdomen, hypertrophy of udder, marked enlargement of the teats pointing downwards and forwards, oedematous swelling of the vulval labiae, formation of bilateral groove on either side of the root of the tail due to sinking caused by relaxation of the sacrosciatic ligaments (Leese, 1927, Prakash and Singh, 1962, Sharma and Vyas, 1970, Musa, 1983, Elias and Cohen, 1986). The females at this stage feel discomfort and keep moving and running aimlessly, if not secured. The mean time for the appearance of premonitory signs of parturition (Table 39) in the camels is quite variable but oedematous swelling of the teats and vulval discharge may be considered as indication for parturition in 2-3 days (Prakash and Singh, 1962, Elias and Cohen, 1986).

Table 39. Average days of appearance of premonitory signs of parturition in camels.

Visible changes	Pre-partum days
Hypertrophy of the mammary gland	24.2 ± 8.3
Appearance of bilateral groove due to relaxation of the sacrosciatic ligament	15.5 ± 2.6
Abdominal distension	12.5 ± 4.2
Oedema of the vulval lips	4.0 ± 1.5
Oedema of the teats	1.5 ± 0.5
Scanty vulval discharge	1.5 ± 0.2

The enlargement of the abdomen of the pregnant females becomes distinct from the non-pregnant animals about 4-6 weeks before the parturition and during the last two weeks, the abdomen is markedly distended. The caudal superficial epigastric vein (milk vein) is consipicuously enlarged and sinusoidal accompanied with the hypertrophy of the udder about 2-3 weeks prior to parturition. In the last week of gestation period, the teats are markedly enlarged due to engorgement with colostrum which may be ejected into streams on application of slight pressure (Prakash and Singh, 1962, Elias and Cohen, 1986).

Parturition in camels is completed in three stages. The observations, so far made show considerable variation in the delineation of three stages of parturition (Leese, 1927, Sharma and Vyas, 1970, Burgemeister, 1975, Moldagaliev, 1976, Chen *et al.*, 1980, Elias and Cohen, 1986). In some recording, the three stages have been made two (Prakash and Singh, 1962) The three stages of parturition are (i) first stage or the period from start of the labour pain to dilatation of the cervix, (ii) second stage or time required for expelling the foetus, and (iii) third stage or duration, of the expu1sion of placenta.

The first stage of labour pain starts with the contraction of uterine musculature forcing the foetus and the fluid with1membranes towards the birth canal. At this time, the female almost stops eating and drinking, rumination becomes irregular and the animal is restless. The tail is either lifted upwards or carried to one side exposing the vulval exit. Frequent micturition in small quantity is common. She looks anxiously on her flank. With the gradual increase intensity of labour pain, the camel becomes more restless and wanders around the pen. If let loose, she keeps on running till the calving starts. At this stage, the females often roll once or twice probably to bring the foetus in dorso-sacral position. This stage lasts for 2 to 10 h in different animals and becomes more intensive in later part. The animal moans and exhibits facial expression of intense pain (Lease, 1927, Prakash and Singh, 1962, Sharma and Vyas, 1970).

Average time from the intensification of the signs of discomfort until the complete dilatation of the cervix is about 95 ± 21 minutes. However, this observation is recorded on small number of females. At the end of this stage, there is pronounced straining due to contractions of the abdominal muscle at the rate of 5.5 ± 1.5 times per 10 minutes. This is accompanied by moans and entrance of the amniochorionic sac into the birth canal (Elias and cohen, 1986). The first water bag appears at the vulva and gradually increases in size and often hangs as a translucent sac or ruptures in the birth canal. At this stage, the head of foetus enters into the birth canal. Straining at this stage coincides with uterine contractions occurring at the rate of 2.5 ± 0.5 (2-3) times in 3 minutes. The digits and nose of the foetus are seen at the vulva. Now most of the female come down on sternum and adopt side posture, forcefully extend limbs to exert pressure through abdominal contraction for expelling the foetus out specially when the foetal chest is leaving the birth canal (Prakash and Singh, 1962). Average time taken for the rupture of water bag is about 7.6 minutes (Sharma and Vyas, 1970). In many cases, amniochorionic sac ruptures in the birth canal and in about 3.5 ± 1.5 minutes of its rupture the foetal nose is seen in the vulva. This is followed by subsequent straining and uterine contractions and takes about 4.5 ± 1.8 minutes for the nose and head to appear in the vulva after the appearance of the nose. The first foreleg slightly preceds the other leg and pushes near the chin in about 6.2 ± 2.1 minutes time and second leg takes about 3.2 ± 0.5 minutes more time. After this the neck of the foetus is expelled in about 11.4 ± 1.5 minutes. This is followed by the expulsion of hump in another 2.6 ± 1.1 minutes and further 2.5 ± 0.5 minutes are required for completing the delivery of foetus. The foetii are mostly expelled out in anterior longitudinal presentation with the head put midway between knees and fetlock joints. The length of umbilical cord is about 25 ± 3.77 cm (Sharma and Vyas, 1970) and it breaks away with the expulsion of foetus or on standing of the mother which stands soon after the birth (Prakash and Singh, 1962).

In the third stage of labour, placenta is expelled out. After expelling the foetus, the female takes short rest for 30-50 (average 38.6 ± 8.5) minutes. After this straining reoccurs at the rate of 2.5 ± 1 per 5 minutes and the expulsion of second water bag or allantochorionic sac takes about 65 ± 4.2 to 146 ± 92 minutes in different camels (Prakash and Singh, 1962, Sharma and Vyas, 1970, Elias and Cohen, 1986) and it is normally expelled intact (Chen and Yuan, 1979). The foetal membrane may also be expelled alongwith the foetus (Singh, 1966). The time taken in different stage of delivery (Table 40) from the on set of the labour pain is highly variable and average duration of parturition has been reported to be about 453 (185-900) minutes (Prakash and Singh, 1962), 282 ± 80 - 356 ± 79 minutes (Sharma and Vyas, 1970), 490 minutes (Musa, 1983) and 374 ± 38 minutes (Elias and Cohen, 1986). Average duration of different stages of delivery in generally much less in nulliparous than the pluriparous camels (Sharma and Vyas, 1970).

Table 40. Average time taken in different stages of parturition (minutes).

Stages of parturition	Mixed herd*	Nulliparous**	Pluriparous**
Number of observations	8	12	51
First stage	275.0 ± 25.0	168 ± 15.6	199.5 ± 49.2
Second stage	33.9 ± 9.0	10.5 ± 4.65	8.4 ± 4.91
Third stage	65.0 ± 4.2	109.9 ± 49.6	146.1 ± 91.1
Total duration	373.9 ± 38.2	281.8 ± 79.6	355.9 ± 79.3

*Elias and Cohen (1986), Sharma and Vyas (1970).

Parturition mostly takes place with the dam in a lateral recumbency but it may also occur in standing position (Gauthier-Pilters, 1959). Average time taken in expelling of the foetus 24 ± 2.34 minutes in dromedary females had been much shorter than 40 ± 2.34 minutes taken by the bactrian females probably due to larger foetus size and double hump in the later animals (Moldagaliev, 1976). A significant variation in parturition duration (second stage) ranging from 8 to 50 minutes (Average 26.8 ± 12 minutes) has been reported in the Chinese bactrian camels (Chen *et al.*, 1980). Scanty lochia is discharged for 12.5 ± 3.5 days post-partum in the camels. The birth normally takes place in the daylight (Elias and Cohen, 1986).

Foetal fluids and membranes

The first water bag is amniochorionic sac which ruptures before expelling the foetus. The fluid amnion is watery and not mucoid as observed in other farm animals (Chen and Yuan, 1979). The second water bag or allantochorionic sac is expelled intact in 65 - 117 minutes after the delivery of foetus. It is partly covered with chorion. The placenta is diffused type involving whole of the chorion and does not contain cotyledons. It is reddish in colour and its outer surface is covered with small red tufted villous processes. The origin of placenta is epidermal and it envelopes the entire foetus except the natural orifices like the lips, anus, umblicus, prepuce in male and vulva in female foetus, teat orifices and also the hooves (Musa, 1979). An extra foetal membrane has been also observed in the camels.

The amniotic fluid is watery and small in quantity. The allantoic fluid is brownish blue and watery in appearance with 1026 ± 0.38 specific gravity and slightly acidic (pH, 6.6 ± 0.1) in reaction. The average weights of allantochorionic sac with fluid 10.3 ± 1.5 kg comprising of 5.3 ± 0.8 kg fluid and 5.6 ± 0.6 kg membranes (Elias and

Cohen, 1986) was different and much less than 21 ± 1.6 kg mean weight of allantochorionic membrane including fluid of Bikaneri camels (Sharma and Vyas, 1970), In another observation, an average 9 litres foetal fluid comprising of about 10-20 per cent amniotic fluid and 80-90 per cent allantoic fluid has been reported in the camels (Musa, 1979).

Hormonal changes during the parturition

A sudden rise in the level of unconjugated oestrogens, 13, 14-dihydro-15-keto-prostaglandin F 2 alpha (PGFM) and corticosteroids is observed which varies during different stages of pre-delivery and delivery period. The concentration of total unconjugated oestrogens in plasma of the pregnant dromedary increases manyfolds from 10-12 pg per ml on day 2-4 before parturition to 203.9 ± 9.35 pg per ml at about 130 minutes and then to 240.9 ± 12.51 pg per ml at 120 minutes and 297.8 ± 3.61 pg per ml at 10 minutes before calving. After the expulsion of foetus, it starts falling abruptly to 268.5 ± 5.63 pg per ml at delivery and reaches as low as 35.2 ± 4.51 pg per ml after 40 minutes post-partum. The pattern of rise and fall is not affected by the sex of foetus in the uterus. The level of PGFM in the blood fluctuates between 200 and 600 pg per ml at about 10 days prior to parturition and then sharply rises to 7.8-10.9 ng per ml at 5.5 hour and then to 13.5 ± 1.16 ng per ml at 5 hours before the delivery. This is followed by further abrupt rise to 38.2 ± 0.67 ng per ml at 60 minutes before and almost similar 39.7 ± 2.47 ng per ml at the time of delivery. The decline is also equally sharp to 29.5 ± 2.04 ng per ml after 10 minutes and to 3.9 ± 0.79 ng per ml at 40 minutes post-partum. The concentration of total plasma corticosteroids is low (3.8 ± 0.51 ng per ml) and remains almost stable during the pre-partum period. However, during parturition, it rises to about 13.3 ± 1.5, 16.9 ± 2.5 and 24.0 ± 3.11 ng per ml at 220 and 110 minutes prior to delivery and at the time of delivery respectively (El-Belaly, 1994).

Post-partum behaviour of the mother

Almost all camels rise immediately after the delivery of foetus but do not lick even if they are pluriparous. They do not even smell or eat the afterbirth unlike other farm animals. Indeed, camel is an excellent mother and shows concern and provides protection to her calf (Matharu, 1966, Elias and Cohen, 1986). Rarely some young nulliparous mother may avoid her calf initially but generally accomodates after human intervention. A mother camel normally does not allow suckling by another calf.

Behaviour of the neo-natal calf

The neo-natal calves quickly adjust with the extra uterine environment. The calf remains for some time near its mother in sternal recumbency. After a short rest of about half an hour, it attempts for rising and acquire standing position in another one hour after several attempts. Thus, the calf stands and establishes locomotion in about two hours of' birth (Prakash and Singh, 1962, Elias and Cohen, 1986). There is an usual natural affinity between the calf and mother. After standing, the calf approaches its mother which then guided it by pushing with her muzzle towards her mammary gland and encourages for suckling. The suckling reflex is observed in one to two hours after parturition. Average time taken for first attempt of suckling is 98.6 ± 11.3 minutes in normal condition and without human assistance. The initial few sucklings are slow and short duration (2-3 minutes) because the calves are not accustomed for suckling. In case of large teats, gentle human assistance may be required initially. The meconium or first faeces is normally passed in 2-3 hours or after the suckling of colostrum and meconium impaction is not observed in camel claves. Foaming of the mouth is normally observed in the calves while suckling but if may also occur in few neonatal calves even before suckling the dam.

The calves begin to respond to auditory stimuli in half an hour of birth and frequent vocalization also occurs. They start primary socialization with the mother after initial suckling in about 125 ± .15 minutes of parturition (Elias and Cohon, 1986). Intense affinity with the nursing person develops in the orphaned calves which are reared on bottle or bucket feeding.

Breeding season in camelids

It is well established that all camelids are seasonal breeder except in areas, where climatic variation is low like coastal areas near equator (Merkt *et al.*, 1990). Some information recorded on breeding season of females which is also rutting period in dromedary males have been compiled (Table 41).

Table 41. Breeding season/months in different camelids.

Species/ location	Breeding months	Source
Dromedary -		
Egypt	December to August	Wilson, 1980
Mali	Feb., March and August-September	
Morocco	May-June	
Pakistan	December to March	
Somalia	April - May	
Sudan	March to August	
Iran	Cold months	Islamy, 1950
India	November to Feb.	Singh and Prakash, 1964
do	January-February	Khan and Kohli, 1973
do	September to Feb.	Sharma and Vyas, 1981
Israel	January to March	Yagil and Etzion, 1980
Coastal tropics	Round the year	Merkt *et al.*, 1990
Saudi Arabia	All months except May, Aug. & Oct.	Arthur *et al.*, 1985.
Not mentioned	November to April	Charnot, 1963
Do	October to January	Kouider *et al.*, 1988
Bactrian -		
China	December to April	Chen *et al.*, 1980
Kazakhasthan	March – April	Barmincev, 1951
do	March – May	Podberezkin, 1951
Alpaca species	April to June	Denneler De La Tour, 1954
Vicuna	March to May	Koford, 1957

Sexual behaviour of male camelids

One-humped camel (*Camelus dromedarius*)

The state of sexual activity in camels is called 'rut' or 'musth'. Rutting is a common feature in male camels, which is normally observed in the active and vigorous male camels during the breeding season but it may persist round the year in some aged bull camels (Williamson and Pyane, 1978). The rutting male is highly passionate, restless and ferocious. It becomes highly mischievious due to intense desire for copulation and tries to break all restraints and often escapes out from the enclosures. There is regular grinding of teeth and frequent expulsion of froathy soft palate which expands into a pinkish balloon like structure and hangs on the side of the Jaw. This is a palatal flap which is blown up due to storage of air in the neck area. Even the docile males turn aggressive and often unapproachable during the rut period. The rutting camels held their head high and legs wide apart with frequent up and down movements of tail. They rarely tolerate rivals. Severe fight among the musth males is quite common in the breeding season and invariably the scrotum is bitten (Singh and Prakash, 1964). The protrusion of palatal flap is accompanied by loud gurgling-roaring. The musth male sudden spreads its hind legs and then sharply brushes his tail against the penis, which is posteriorly directed. After 4-5 beats, the tail is held under the urethral opening. A small amount of urine deposited on the tail is splashed onto the back. This action is repeated 3-5 times per hour. After few days, the back of male is caked with vile smelling dried crust (Yagil and Etzion, 1980). The animal is thrown into persipiration and profuse discharge of secretion from the poll glands which become prominent. Shortly the male swallows the flap and attains normal condition. Such fits recur it intervals of 15-30 minutes and lasts for the entire rutting season (Sharma and Vyas, 1981) The secretion of poll glands is brown watery emitting characteristic strong odour (Matharu, 1966, Fraser, 1968). Testoesterone content is very high in this fluid (approximately 36 ng per ml) and equal to that in the blood (Yagil and Etzion, 1979).

A ferocious fight is inevitable when more than one musth male comes together. The weaker camels are forced by the strongest one to suppress their sexual desire (Singh, 1966). The voluntary suppression of sexual desire is related to the status of the male in the hierarchy of the herd (Fraser, 1968). This is a purely psychological response developed due to fear in young and weaker males.

It becomes difficult to use the rutting males for work and riding becomes risky (Singh and Prakash, 1964). However, some owners of riverine type baggage camels use their rutting males for carrying pack loads after applying a strong muzzle and controlling their aggressiveness by whipping (Unpublished observations, N.N. Pathak). The rutting males loose their appetite and may suffer from non-specific diarrhoea occassioally. More passionate males, desirous of mating any female whether in heat or not, develop wind sucking habit which causes continuous belching. They gurgle and produce large amount of milky froath almost continuously. However, sexual desire can be considerably suppressed by overworking to tiredness.

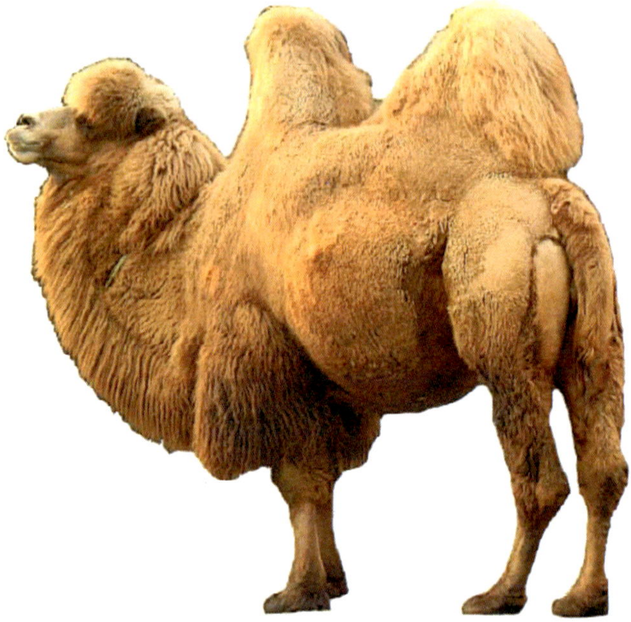

Double-humped camel

Double-humped camel (*Camelus bactrianus*)

Sexual behaviour or bactrian males is more or less similar to that of dromedary males. But, bactrian male does not blow soft palate (Cauvet, 1926). Average sexual activities in bactrian males have been measured to be about 3.65 + 0.54 on a 5 points scale and it varies with the change in age and vigour of the animal (Rakhimzhanov, 1975).

New world Camelids or Llamoids

All llamoid species except the guanco are tamed animals reared on grazing at high lands. They are generally kept in large size flocks. Each eligible mature male maintains a drove or harm of 5-15 breedable females and their young progeny. Young males are expelled out from the group on the onset of puberty at 8-12 months of age. Expelled young males unite in flocks of 20 to 100 or more and lead isolated life (Dennler De La Tour, 1954). Well grown energetic males subsequently form their own drove by eloping females from the old harams or by acquiring young females.

Sexual behaviour of female camelids

Dromedary females

The females in oestrus like the company of potent male until they conjugate and conceive. A female in heat strongly resists her separation from the male and often sits down, when forcibly driven away for working or riding (Singh and Prakash, 1964). In the beginning of oestrus, the female becomes restless and off feed for first one or two days which gradually subsides towards the end of oestrus. A female in heat comes near the male emitting soft rhythmic grunting sound. The tail is either raised high or deviated to side exposing the moist and somewhat swollen vulva. Frequent micturition in small quantity is quite common (Joshi *et al.*, 1978, Musa, 1979). The young females reared alone away from the males jump and run away in the field on the onset of oestrus and wander in search of male (Joshi *et al.*, 1978).

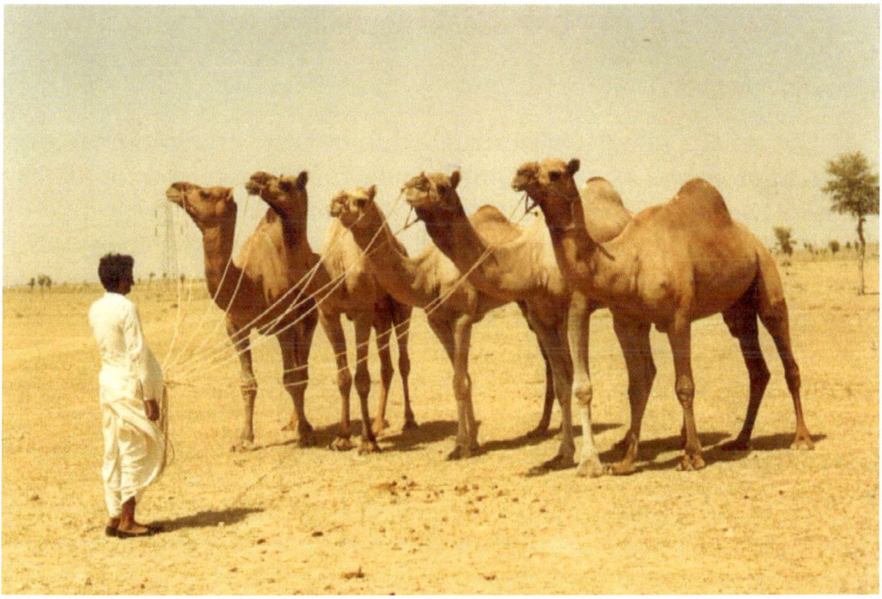

Dromedary camel (Bharat)

Bactrian females

The sexual behaviour is similar to that in dromedary females. The intensity of sexual behaviour is quite variable and high during the longer day length.

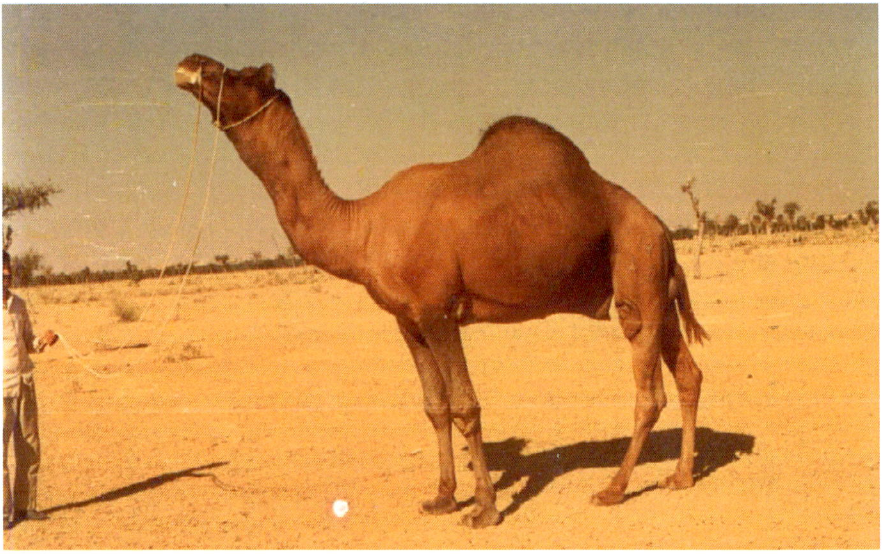

Dromadory Stand in rut

Llamoid females

The alpaca female in oestrus exhibits very strange behaviour. When approached by a male, the female quickly assumes copulatory posture (ventral decubitus). Almost all females in the flock may be found to be sexually receptive at the same time (Fernandez Baca, 1975). The females are generally restless and move close to male pushing him frequently to attract and excite for mating. When many female Llamoids come in heat at the same time, some of them often desert their mate to join a new mate preferably from the isolated bachelors.

Courtship in camels

The male camel is capable to detect the female in oestrus which is then driven out of the herd. The rutting male approaches the females in breeding season and smells their external genitalia and groin. After this, the male extends his head and neck upwards with upward drawn upper lip baring the teeth i.e., the exhibition of Flehman reaction. Some males take 2-3 rounds of the female in heat, become aggressive and bite the female in her genital region and on the hump and back of the neck often causing open bleeding wounds. At this stage, the male is extremely restless. The ballooned dulaa is protruded out with commanding roaring. Now the male forces the female to squat for mating. Sometimes, a female in oestrus approaches the rutting male.

She comes near the male, moves in front, rubs her hind parts against the male, holds her tail upwards or towards a side and passes urine in small amounts but doest not submit easily. Once the male is excited, she runs away when chased by the male (Khan and Kohli, 1973, Hartley, 1979).

In penned females, when the male teaser is brought near a female in oestrus, she shows affinity for him and sniffs his external genitalia, prepuce and anal region. She comes in close proximity of the teaser bull and bites on the face, muzzle and ears of the male. She twists her neck around the neck of the teaser. Shortly both partners come close to each other and remain in head to head position for some time. After this the female adopts a sitting posture exposing her vulva by driving her tall towards a side or upwards. The female remains in such position for some time even when teaser is removed (Joshi *et al.*, 1980).

Llamoids

The males take active part in mating. They detect the female in oestrus and approach for mating. A female in heat does not resist or engage in pre-coital courtship rather assumes copulatory posture quickly. Almost all females in a drove become receptive at the same time and surround the mating couple.

Mating (copulation / coitus) in camels

The act of copulation in camels has been closely observed by several workers (Singh and Prakash, 1964, Khan and Kohli, 1973, Joshi *et al.*, 1980, Sharma and Vyas, 1981, Cristofori *et al.*, 1986). The passionate camels do not care for the presence of strangers and copulate immediately (Gauthier-Pilters, 1974). Other females in oestrus gather near the copulating couple and watch the act eagerly. Some females in intense heat may bite the ear of copulating male and remain near them waiting for her turn (Yasin and Wahid, 1957, Joshi *et al.*, 1980).

Copulation in camels takes place in sitting posture facing in the same direction and not in tail to tail position, as commonly believed due to posterior direction of the external genitalia in the males. During mating, the female keeps on sitting normally while the male adopts a dog sitting posture with hind limbs flexed and resting on the ground from the heels to the hock. The stifle almost touches the ground. The forelegs are extended on each side in front of the shoulder of the female hold tasting foot in her shoulder depression to form a firm grip of the female.

On initial penetration of the penis, there is a sudden contraction of the abdominal muscles particularly the rectus abdominis muscle, as a result of which the pelvic region of the male is quickly brought into direct opposition to the external genitalia of the female and intromission is completed. The male locates the vulvar opening by rotating the erect penis on its longitudinal axis. Consequent upon the complete penetration, there is voluminous froathing and gurgling noise from the male while the female grunts. During the act of copulation, some females bite the stud on his face, neck and legs and emitted a peculiar type of grunting sound. The male camel, unlike horse stallion and cattle bull makes penile strokes in this position, when all the joints of his back legs are flexed. After ejaculation the muscles of the hind legs contract, respiration increases, the male stands on hind legs and discount the female. There is a marked sex drive and short preparatory stage. A marked coordination in balancing the body on mounting, grasping the female, searching the vulvar opening and the penile strokes ending in ejaculation are observed in the male camel (Singh and Prakash, 1964, Joshi *et al.,* 1980). In a single mating period, the male may ejaculate three to four times, but each service starts by fresh penile penetration (Hartley, 1979). Normally males do not need help in penetration but also do not mind if assisted, which reduces the time of searching the vulvar opening and save the male from exhausting during copulation.

Mating in llamoids

The males are very active and often aggressive during the copulation. The male alpacas show remarkable mating activity, when put into a flock of the females. During first 3 days, the males are involved in intense copulatory activity which declines considerably inspite of the presence of receptive females. However, on shifting to a new flock of females, they resume their sexual activity (Fernandez Baca *et al.,* 1972). Like camels, in llamoid females also copulation takes place in the prone posture.

Duration of copulation in camelids

A great variation has been found in the duration of copulation among the different species of camelids which is generally shorter in large species like bactrian and dromedary camel and longer in small size llamoids. Whole day intermittent sexual activity in dromedary has been reported in earlier literature (Leonard, 1994). An hour long mating activity has been also reported on hear say basis (Droandi, 1915). Some of the observations on copulation duration in different species have been compiled (Table 42).

Table 42. Copulation duration in different camelids.

Species	Copulation duration (minutes)	Source
Bactrian camel	12.15 ± 0.94	Rakhimzhanov, 1975
do	2-4	Chen *et al.*, 1980
Dromedary camel	11.4 (7-21)	Singh & Prakash, 1964
do	24.13 ± 0.4 (21-27)	Joshi *et al.*, 1980
do	10 (8-15)	Sharma & Vyas, 1981
do	5.6 ± 2.25	Rai *et al.*, 1988
Alpaca	30	Cuilbridge & Moro, 1965
do	20-50	Fenandez Baca, 1975

References

Abdel-Rahim, S.E., Abdel-Rahim, K. and El-Nazier, A.E. 1994. Production and reproduction of one-humped camels in the Al-Quasim region, Saudi Arabia. J. Arid Environ., 26 : 53.

Abdel-Raouf, M. and El-Naggar, M. 1964. Studies on reproduction in camel (Camelus dromedaries). 1. Mating. UAR J. Vet. Sci., 1:113.

Abdel-Raouf, M. and El-Naggar, M. 1978. Studies on reproduction in camel (Camelus dromedaries). VI. Properties and constituents of ejaculated semen. Proc. VIIIth Intern., Cong. Anim. Reprod. And Arti. Insem. Cracow.

Abdel-Raouf, M. Fateh El-Bab, M.R. and Owaida, M.M. 1975. Studies on reproduction in camel (Camelus dromedaries). J. Reprod. Fertil., 43: 109.

Abdo, M.S., Al-jahabi, A.S. and Al-Kawafi, A.A. 1968. Studies on the ovaries of the female camel during the reproductive cycle and in condition affected by cysts. Cornell Vet., 59 : 418.

Ali, H.A., Tingari, M.D. and Moniem, K.A. 1978. On the morphology and histochemistry of the ampulla doctus deferentis of the camel (Camelus dromedaries). J. Anat., 125 : 277.

Arthur, G.H., A. Rahim, A.T. and Al-Hindi, A.S. 1985.

Aueljbekov, K. 1967. Camel breeding : A profitable field. Konevod. Konnyi. Sport, 5 : 6.

Barmintsev, V. 1951. Rectal examination of the reproductive organs of the camel. Konevod. Konnyi. Sport, 1 : 138.

Beniwal, B.K. and Chaudhry, A.L. 1983. Growth pattern in Bakaneri camel (Camelus dromedaries). Indian J. Anim. Sci., 53 : 101.

Bhargava, K.K., Sharma, V.D. and Singh, M. 1965. A study of the birth weight and body measurements of camel (Camelus dromedaries). Indian J. Vet. Sci. Anim. Husb., 35 : 358.

Blagovescenskii, V. 1963. Reserves in the production of milk and meat. Konevod. Konnyi. Sport, 33 (10) : 8.

Bodenheimer, Bosaev, J. 1938. Sexual activity of camels and organization of service. Konevod. Konnyi Sport, 8 : 26.

Bravo, W. and Sumar, J. 1989. Laproscopic examination of the ovarian activity in alpaca. Anim. Reprod. Sci., 21 : 271.

Cauvet, C.D.T. 1926. Le chameau. 947 pp. Bailliere, Paris.

Chaharasbi, H., Radmehr, B. and Goulbarzhagh, F. 1975. Anatomy and history of the reproductive organs of the Iranian camel (Camelus dromedaries). J. Vet. Fac., Uni., Tehran, 30:42.

Charnot, Y. 1958. Repercussion de la deshydration sur la biochimie et l'endocrinologie du dromedaire. Thesis, Faculte des Sciences, Paries.

Charnot, Y. 1963a. Synchronisation of growth of the palatal expansion and the testis during the sexual cycle in the dromedary. Bull. Soc. Nat. Physiol., Maroc., 43 : 49.

Charnot, Y. 1963b. Sexual endocrinology and dehydration in the male dromedary. C.R. Seanc. Soc. Biol., 159 : 1103.

Charnot, Y. 1964. Le cycle testicular du dromedaire. Bull. Soc. Nat. Physiol., Maroc, 44 : 37.

Charnot, Y. and Racadot, 1963.

Chapman, M.J. 1985. Mongolia : Bactrian camel. Worls Anim. Rev., 55:14.

Chen, B.X. and Yuan, Z.X. 1979. Reproductive pattern of the bactrian camel. Proc. IFS intern. Symp. Camels, Sudan, p. 251.

Chen, B.X. and Yuan, Z.X. 1980. Reproductive pattern of the bactrian camel. Proc. IFS Gangsu Agril. Uni., China.

Chen, B.X. and Yuan, Z.X. 1984. Reproductive pattern of the bactrian camel. In: The Camelid: An all purpose animal (Ed. W.R. Cockrail). Vol. 1. Scandinavian Inst. of African studies, Uppsala, Sweden, p. 364.

Chen, P.M., Kang, C.L., Yuan, Z.X. and Ge, Y.G. 1980. Reproductive pattern of the bactrian camel. Acta Vet. et Zootech, 11:60-146 and 12:85 (1981)

Chen, B.X., yuan, Z.X. and Pan, G.w. 1985. Semen induced ovulation in the bactrian camel (Camelus bactrianus). J. reprod. Fertil., 73:335.

Chowdhary, B. 1986. Some important biological and production characters of the Bikaneri camel. Indian J. Anim. Prod. Mange., 2:145.

Cristofori, P., Aria, G., Seren, E., Bono, G., Anden, A. and Nur, H.M. 1986. Somalia: endocribiological aspects of reproduction in the female camel. World Anim. Rev., 57:22.

Dahl, G. and Hjort, A. 1976. Having herds: pastoral herd growth and household economy. University of Stockholm, Sweden.

Degan, A.A. and Lee, D.G. 1982. The male genital tract of the dromedary (one-humped) camel. Zentralb. Vet. med. Reihe C, 11:267.

Dennler de la Tour, G. 1971. Inheritance of the hump in the camel, dromedary and camel X dromedary cross. Anim. Breed Abst., 40:364.

Droandi, I.K. 1976. Milk production and fat percentage and their inheritance in bactrian camel, dromedary and hybrids. Izvestiya Akademii Nauk Kazakhskoi, SSR, Seriya Biolog., 14(6) : 69 (Anim. Breed. Abst., 1979, 47:483).

El-Belely, M.S. 1994. Endocrine changes with emphasis on 13, 14-dihydro-15-keto-prostaglandin F 2 a and cortico-steroids, before and during parturition in dromedary camels (Camelus dromedarius). J. agric. Sci., Camb., 122:315.

Elias, E. and Cohen, D. 1986. Parturition in the camel (Camelus dromedarius) and some behavioural aspects of their newborn. Comp. Biochem. Physiol. 84A:413.

Elias, E., Bedrak, E. and Cohen, D. 1985. Induction of oestrus in the camel (Camelus dromedarius) during seasonal anoestrus. J. Reprod. Fertil., 74:519.

El-Manna, M.M., Tingari, M.D. and Ahmed, A.K. 1986. Studies on camel semen. II. Biochemical characteristics. Anim. Reprod. Sci., 12:223.

El-Wishy, A.B. and Omar, A.M. 1975. On the relation between testes size and sperm reserves in the one-humped camel (Camelus dromedarius). Beitr. Trop. Landwrit. Vet. med., 13:391.

El-Wishy, A.B., Hemeida, N.A., Omar, M.A., Mobarak, M.A. and El-Sayed, M.A.I. 1981. Functional changes in the pregnant camel with special reference to foetal growth. British Vet. J., 137:527.

England, Barry G., Foote, W.C., Cardozo, Armendo G., Mathews, D.H. and Riera, Simon. 1971. Oestrus and mating behaviour in the llama (Llama glama). Animal Behaviour, 19:722.

Fernandez-Baca, S. 1970. Luteal function and the nature of reproductive failure in the alpaca. Ph.D thesis. Cornell Univ., Ithaca, USA.

Fernandez-Baca, S. 1972 (1971). The alpaca : reproduction and breeding. Anim. Breed. Abst., 40:366.

Fernandez Baca, S. 1975. Alpaca breeding in the high Andes. World Animal Rev., 14:1.

Fernandez Baca, S. 1993. Manipulation of reproductive functions in male and female New World Camelids. Anim. Reprod. Sci., 33:307.

Fernandez Baca, S., Madden, D.H.L. and Novoa, C. 1970. Effects of different mating stimuli on induction of ovulation in the alpaca. J. Reprod. Fertil., 22:261.

Fernandez Baca, S., Novoa, C. and Sumar, J. 1972. Actividad reproductive en la alpaca mantenida en separacion del macho. ALP A Mem., 7:7.

Fernandez Baca, S., Sumar, J., Novoa, C. and Leyva, V. 1973. Relacion entre la ubicacion del cuerpo luteo y la localizacion del embrion en la alpaca. Rev. Inv. Pec. (IVITA) University, San Marcos, 2:131.

Fraser, A.F. 1968. Reproductive behaviour in ungulates. 202 pp. Academic Press, London.

Gauthier-Pilters, H. 1959. Einige Beobachtungen zum Droh-, Angriffsund Kampfverhalten des Dromedarhongstes, sowie uber Geburt und Verhaltensentiwicklung des. Jungtieres in her nordwest-lichen Sahara. Z. Tierpsychol., 16:593.

Gauthier-Pilters, H. 1974. The behaviour and ecology of camels in the Sahara with special reference to nomadism and water management. ICUN Pub., New Ser., 2 (24): 542.

Goswami, S.K., Singh, Yashwant and Nagpal, S.K. 1994. Histology of the ductus epididymidis in camel and histology and histochemical studies in ductus deferens of camel: non-glandular part. Indian J. Anim. Sci., 64:230 & 1328.

Guilbridge, P.D.L. and Moro, S.M. 1965. Animal health at high altitude. Veterinarian, Oxford, 3:33.

Gupta, A.K., Chowdhary, M.S. and Barhat, N.K. 1978. A note on optimum time for service in camel (Camelus dromedarius). Indian J. Anim. Sci., 48:324.

Hartley, B.J. 1979. The dromedary of the horn of Africa. Proc. Workshop on camels (IFS, Stockholm), Khartoum, Ethiopia.

Hira, L.M. 1947. Camel breeding in India. Indian Farming, 8:504.

Islamy, A. 1950. Riding camels around Khas and Iranshahr. Rev. Fac. Med. Vet., Tehran, 12:187.

Iwema, S. 1960. the ship of the desert. Veeteelt. en 2nd Zuivelberichten, 3:390.

Joshi, C.K., Pareek, P.K. and Vyas, K.K.. Note on the sexual behaviour of she camel during oestrus. Indian J. Anim. Sci., 50:588.

Joshi, C.K., Vyas, K.K. and Pareek, K.K. 1978. Studies on oestrus cycle in Bikaneri she camel. Indian J. Anim. Sci., 48:141.

Kamoun, M. and Wilson, T. 1994. Improving early reproduction characteristic of Tunisian camels by nutritional and management interventions. J. Arid Environ., 26:89.

Khan, A.K. and Kohli, I.S. 1973. A note on biometrics of the camel's spermatozoa. Indian J. Anim. Sci., 43:792.

Khanna, N.D., Tandon, S.N. and Rai, A.K. 1990. Breeding parameters of Indian camels. Indian J. Anim. Sci., 60:1347.

Koford, C.B. 1957. The vicuna and the puna. Ecol. Monogr., 27:153.

Kouider, S., Ateeq, G. and Kolb, E. 1988. Stuides on the content of total protein, urea, total fat, cholesterol and bilirubin in blood plasma of camels during the course of a year. Monatshfte fur Vet. med., 43:139.

Leese, A.S. 1927. A treatise on the one-humped camel in health and disease. 382 pp. Haynes and Sons, Stanford Line.

Leonard, A.G. 1894. The camel: Its uses and management. 335. Longman, Green and Co., London.

Lesbre, F.X. 1906. Precis d'exterieur du cheval et des principaux mamiferes domestiques. Asselin et Houzeau, Paris.

Mares, R.G. 1954. Animal husbandry, animal industry and animal disease in the Somaliland protectorate. British Vet. J., 110:411.

Marie, M. and Anouassi, A. 1986. Mating induced luteinizing hormone surge and ovulation in the female camel (Camelus dromedarius). Biol. Reprod., 35:792.

Matharu, B.S. 1966. Animal management: Camel care. Indian Farming, 16(7):19.

Meredov, B. 1984. Some problems of camel breeding in Turkmenia. Konevod. Konnyi. Sport, 12:22.

Mehta, V.S., Anand Prakash, A.H. and Singh, M. 1962. gestation period in camels. Indian vet. J., 39:387.

Merkt, H., Rath, D., Musa, B. and El-Naggar, M.A. 1990. The penis and prepuce of the one-humped camel (Camelus dromedarius). Zentbl. Vet. med., 19:787.

Moldagaliev, T.M. 1976. The effect of foetal size and pelvic measurements on parturition in different species of camel. Anim. Breed. Abstr., 44:653.

Musa, B.E. 1979. The development, presentation, position and posture of the foetus in camel (Camelus dromedarius). Sudan J. Vet. Sci. Anim. Husb., 20:37.

Musa, B.E. 1983. Normal parturition in the camel (Camelus dromedarius). Vlaams Diergenee. Tijdschrift, 52:255.

Musa, B.E. and Abu Sineina, M.E. 1976. Some observations on reproduction in the female camel. Acta Vet., Yogoslo., 26:63.

Musa, B.E. and Abu Sineina, M.E. 1978. The oestrus cycle of the camel (Camelus dromedarius). Vet. Rec., 103:556.

Musa, B.E., Merkt, H., Sieme, H. Hago, B.E.D. and Hoppen, H.O. 1990. The female camel (Camelus dromedarius) and the artificial insemination. Proc. Unite de coordination pour l'elevage Camelin, paris, p. 257.

Nagpal, S.K., Sudhakar, L.S., Singh, G. and Singh, Y. 1987. Gross and histomorphological observations on the penis of camel. Indian J. Anim. Sci., 57:671.

Nanda, P.N. 1966. Management of camels. Indian Farming, 15(12):38.

Nawito, M., Shalash, M.R., Hoppe, R. and Rakha, A.M. 1967. Reproduction in female camel. Bull. Nat. Res. Center, Cairo No. 2.

Novoa, C. 1970. Reproduction in camelidae, Review. J. Reprod. Fertil., 22:3.

Novoa, C., Sumar, J., Leyva, V. and Fernandez-Baca, S. 1973. Incremento reproductivo en alpaca de explotaciones comerciales mediante metode de empadre alternado. Rev. Inv. Pec. (IVITA), Univ. San Marcos, Lima, 2:191.

Osman, A.M. and El-Azab, E.A. 1974. Conadal-epididymal sperm reserves in the camel (Camelus dromedarius). J. Reprod. Fertil., 38:425.

Osman, D.I. 1986. The intratesticular ducts of the camel (Camelus dromedarius). Anim. Reprod. Sci., 10:47.

Osman, D.I., Moniem, K.A. and Tingari, M.D. 1979. Histological observations on the testis of the camel with special emphasis on spermatogenesis. Acta Anot., 104:164.

Osman, D.I. and Ploen, K. 1986. (i) Spermatogenesis in the camel. (ii) Fine structures of the Sertoli cells in the camel. (iii) Fine structure of epididymal spermatozoa in the camel, Camelus dromedarius. Anim. Reprod. Sci., 10:23, 37, 177.

Pareek, P.K., Joshi, C.K. and Vyas, K.K. 1981. Note on the biometry of genital organs of female camel (Camelus dromedarius). Indian J. Anim. Sci., 51:1010.

Parkes, A.S. 1969. Marshall's physiology and reproduction. 3rd ed. Longman, London.

Podberezkin, J.A. 1951. Experience of the work of a better camel breeding farm. Konevod. Konnyi Sport, 10:42.

Prakash, A. Singh, V. 1962. Normal parturition in camels. Indian vet. J., 39:551.

Rakhimzhanov, G.R. 1975. The evaluation of sexual reflexes in male bactrian camels. Referativnyi Zhurnal, 9.58.398.

San Martin, M. 1961

San Martin, M., Copiara, M., Zumiga, J., Rodriguez, R., Bustinza, G. and Acosta, L. 1968. Aspects of reproduction in the alpaca. J. Reprod. Fertil., 16:395.

Shalash, M.R. 1965. Some reproductive aspects in the female camel. World Rev. Anim. Prod., 4:103.

Shalash, M.R. and Nawito, M. 1963. Sterility in female camels. Dtscb. Tierarztil. Wochenschr., 70:522.

Sharma, S.S. and Vyas, K.K. 1971. Peculiar antipartum characteristic behaviour in single-humped camel (Camelus dromedarius). Haryana Vet., 10:59.

Sharma, S.S. and Vyas, K.K. 1981. Studies on sexual physiology of stud camel (Camelus dromedarius). Indian vet. J., 58:743.

Shri Ram, Singh, Balbir and Dhanda, O.P. 1977. A note on genetic studies on gestation length, birth weight and intra-uterine development index in Indian camel (Camelus dromedarius). Indian vet. J., 54:953.

Singh, H. 1966. Camel care. Intensive Agric., January, p. 9.

Singh, U.B. and Bhardwaj, M.B. 1980. Histological studies on the testicular seminal pathway and change in the epididymis of the camel (Camelus dromedarius). Acta Anat., 108:481.

Strain, M.G. and Strain, S.S. 1987. Caring for the premature llama. Vet. Med., 82:1243.

Sumar, J. and Garcia, M. 1986. Fisiologia de la reproduction de la alpaca. In: Nuclear and related techniques in Anim. Prod. Health. IAEA, Vienna, p. 149.

Sumar, J., Novoa, C. and Fernandez-Baca, S. 1972. Fisiologia reproductive post-partum en la alpaca. Rev. Inv. Pec. (IVITA), Univ. San Marcos, Lima, 1:21.

Tayeb, M.A.F. 1948. Trans. Blin, P.C. L'appareil genital male du chameau. Rev. Elev. Med. Vet. Pays Trop., 4:157.

Tayeb, M.A.F. 1953. Trans. Blin, P.C. les organes genitaux de la chamelle. Rev. Elec. Med. Vet. Pays Trop., 1:17.

Terentjev, S.M. 1951. Experience in stud work on a camel breeding farm. Konevod. Konnyi Sport, 11:20.

Terentjev, S.M. 1963. Camel breeding in Astarkhan province. Zivotnovodstvo, 25:54.

Tingari, M.D., El-Manna, M.M., Rahim, A.T.A., Ahmed, A.K. and Hamad, M.H. 1986. Stuides on camel semen. I. Electro-ejaculation and some aspects of semen characteristics. Anim. Reprod. Sci., 12:213.

Tingari, M.D. and Moneim, K.A. 1979. On the regional histology and histochemistry of the epididymis of the camel (Camelus dromedarius). J. Reprod. Fertil., 57:11.

Tingari, M.D., Moneim, K.A. and Kunzel, E. 1979. Observations on the fine structure of the testicular interstitial cells in the camel (Camelus dromedarius). Q.J. Exp. Physiol., 64:39.

Vorano, A.E. and Bertoni, J.A. 1984. Biological and production parameters in the llama (Cuvier) on natural pastures of the high Andean Plateau, with supplementation and different stocking rates. Rev. Argentina de Prod. Anim., 4:325.

Vyas, A.P. 1985. Camel breeding in desert. Transactions of Indian Soc. Desert Technol. 10: 1.(Anim. Breed. Abstr., 1987, 55:68).

Williamson, G. and Payne, W.J. A 1978. An Introduction to Animal Husbandry in the Tropics. Longman, Singapore.

Watson, R.M. 1969. A census of the domestic stock of North Eastern Province Kenya. Mimeo, Nairobi, 135 pp.

Wilson, R.T. 1978. Studies on the livestock of Souther Darfur, Sudan. 5. Notes on camels. Trop. Anim. Hlth. Prod., 10:19.

Wilson, R.T. 1984. The camel. Longman, London.

Wilson, R.T. 1986. Reproductive performance and survival of young one-humped camels on Kenya commercial ranges. Anim. Prod., 42:375.

Yagi, R. and Etzion, Z. 1979. Seasonal changes in hormones and behaviour in the male camel. Refuah Vet., 36:70.

Yagil, R. and Etzion, Z. 1980. Hormonal and behavioural pattern in the male camel (Camelus dromedarius). J. Reprod. Fertil., 58:61.

Yagil, R. and Etzion, Z. 1984. Enhanced reproduction in camels (Camelus dromedarius). Comp. Biochem. Physiol., 79A:201.

Yasin, S.A. and Wahid, A. 1957. Pakistan camels- a preliminary survey. Agric. Pakistan, 8:289.

□□□

Chapter 5

The Mammary Glands, Milk and Milk Products

The Mammary Glands of Dromedary or One-humped Camel

The mammary gland is a modified cutaneous gland which is found functional in females. The development of the mammary glands is closely linked with the growth and functions of the genital organs of the females. Hence, mammary gland is considered as an accessory sex organ. The mammary glands together are called the udder. The udder is placed in the inguinal region in all species of camel and cameloides. The udder is non-functional and rudimentary in the males.

The udder of the dromedary (Camelus dromadarius) is made of four quarters encapsulated in a soft and pliable cutaneous pouch. Each quarter of the udder is an independent unit separated from each other with a distinct connective tissue septum. The udder in camels is normally disc shaped. The gland of each quarter drains through its short finger shaped test (Osman and Ismail, 1988).

External structure of the udder

The udder is contained in a pouch of skin which is thin, lightly pigmented and pliable. The skin contains large number of 'sebaceous and sweat glands. The development of the udder starts actively with the functional development of the sex glands with the onset of puberty and the glands are fully developed before the parturition and milk secretion normally starts at calving.

Internal structure of the udder

The gland of each quarter is made of parenchyma, connective tissue, stroma, ducts and alveolar system. Each gland is separated into several lobules by connective tissue septa. Individual 1obules are separated by a special arrangement of connective tissue which surrounds the lobules and called interlobular connective tissue. Thin strands of connective tissue as intralobular connective tissue penetrate inside the lobules which surround the alveoli and the intralobular ducts. The intralobular connective tissue is characterised by its delicate structure compared with that present in rest of the mammary gland.

The duct system begins with small intralobular ducts. The lumen of the small intralobular duct is lined with low simple secretary epithelium which becomes columnar in the large ducts. The epithelial cells are arranged on a distinct basement membrane.

The acini or alveoli are small vesicles of unequal size and together they form the alveolar system of the lobule. The flattened to columnar epithelial lining of the alveoli greatly vary with the secretary activity of the gland. Numerous blood capillaries and a few fat cells are found in the interlobular connective tissue and surround the alveoli (Nosier, 1973).

Internal structure of the involuted mammary gland

Involution of the mammary glands occur in the pregnant and non-pregnant lactating females. During involution, regression of the parenchymatous tissue occurs and the interstitial connective tissue is filled in the spaces formed, by reduction of the alveoli. The volume of lobule is also reduced significantly. With the progress in the lactation period, there is a gradual loss of gland and secretary activity causing considerable reduction in the volume of the lobule. The ratio in the areas of glandular and non-glandular tissues is usually 2:1 in the lactating and 0.36:1 in the non-lactating tissue (Nosier, 1973). In sudanese camels, the volume of udder is 1783 cm; and 655 cm; glandular tissue 79.32 and 23.85% and connective tissue 13.19 and 69.01 per cent structure of the teats (Papilla mammae) respectively (Ibrahim *et al.,* 1988).

The teats of dromedary camels are short, narrow and cylindrical but slightly tapering towards the apex. The occurrence of any supranummerary teat has not been recorded even after examining 200 udders. The average size of all the four teats in a udder is more or less similar but a large variation has been observed due to age and lactation number (Table 43). Each teat possesses two and sometimes three cistern which are completely separated from each other. Each cistern or lactiferous simus is spindle shaped which tapers distally and continues into the streak canal. The streak canals open normally in a common small pouch formed near the apex of the teat, but in some animals the streak canals open directly on the surface of the apex of the teat.

Table 43. Size of the teats of dromedary camel.

Measurements (cm)	Right teat		Left teat	
	Range	Mean	Range	Mean
Length, fore teat	1.6 - 4.0	2.38	1.6 - 4.0	2.40
rear teat	1.5 - 3.1	2.41	1.2 - 3.3	2.38
Diameter, fore teat-				
at base	0.9 - 2.3	1.40	0.9 - 2.3	1.50
at apex	0.3 - 1.3	0.60	0.2 - 1.1	0.53
rear teat-				
at base	0.8 - 2.4	1.50	1.0 - 2.2	1.50
at apex	0.4 - 1.0	0.60	0.4 - 1.8	0.62

Source: Saleh *et al.* (1971).

The cutaneous layer of the teats contains few hair follicles but these are entirely absent at the apex. The hair follicles are associated with sebaceous glands at the base of the teats but no sweat glands. Faint pigmentation is restricted to the stratum germinativum. Just below the cutaneous layer, a thick layer of fibromuscular vascular tissues is present, which is formed of dense connective tissue with smooth muscle fibre bundles arranged circularly and longitudinally. At the middle and apex of the teat, the circular muscle fibres predominate and completely encircle the two (rarely three) teat cisterns. At the apex of the teat, these fibres form the teat sphincter.

The blood vessels are mainly longitudinal and tortuous. Many elastic fibres are present in the dense connective tissue of the dermis and also in the fibromuscular vascular layer.

The teat cisterns are lined by two layers of columnar cells. The streak canal is lined by stratified squamous epithelium, which is keratinised in some parts. The streak canals open into a common small pouch lined with the same keratinised epithelium as occurs in the apex of the teat. Keratin probably provides protection against the microbial infection and reduces the incidence of mastitis. The mucous membrane of the teat cistern possesses a number of slightly elevated longitudinal folds but no transverse folds or pockets. The absence of pockets in the teat cistern may also provide protection against the infection lowering the incidence of mastitis. (Saleh *et al.*, 1971).

Shape and size of the udder and teats of bactrian camel

The udder of bactrian camels is either round and smoth or somewhat furrowed due to well-defined and prominent septa of the four quarters. The measurements of the udder and teats (Table 44) differ due to structure in mature camels (Belokobylenko and Musaev, 1982). Physical treatment influences the size of the udder and teat as twice daily massage of udder and teats about one and half months before the expected date of calving increased their size, 1982).

Table 44. Size of the udder and teats of Bactrian camels

Measurements (cm)	Round udder	Quarters defined udder	Twice daily massage of udder	No massage of udder
Udder –				
Circumference	68.5	70.5	65.1	58.7
Depth	15.0	13.5	20.0	17.4
Teats –				
Length, fore teat	2.97	2.92	1.5	1.3
rear teat	3.24	3.58	1.4	1.1
Circumference –				
fore teats	8.45	7.50	4.6	4.4
rear teats	8.40	9.00	4.5	4.6
Distance between				
fore teats	19.3	18.3	14.6	14.8
rear teats	11.0	9.5	7.3	8.4

The udder of adult females of several lactation is larger than the udder of the first calvers in circumference but not in depth. Massaging of udder for 5-6 weeks before calving increases the size of udder and length of teats without affecting the circumference of teats and their placement on the udder Musaev, 1982).

The structure of udder and its volume have some relation with milk yield which has been found higher in camels with rounded udder in cmparison to those with well demarkted quarters. However, the shape of udder does not affect the milking time (Belokobylenko and Musaev, 1982). The udder of different Lama sp also contains four mammary glands each having one teat (Fernandes Baca, 1975).

Let down of milk and milking

Both hand milking and machine milking methods are used for the milking of dromedary and bactrian camels. Presence as well as suckling by the calf is required for the let down of milk. Like cow calf, the camel calf also suckle left side. Initially, the calf changes the teats quickly but soon starts to suckle one teat continuously unless changed by the milker or milk flow rate is decreased. A few butting like that of cow calf is also observed in camel calf. In case of calf death, lactation ceases unless a foster calf is accepted or the mother is conditioned mostly by beating to inflict more pain making her to forget the calf. Other methods to stimulate the let down of milk are the use of the skin of dead calf on the body of another calf (Mares, 1954) or making dummy calf by stuffing the skin of dead calf as in the case of buffaloes (Pathak, 1992). Most of the females accept the calf of another female for the let down of milk (Cossins, 1971). Let down time is normally less than one minute.

In bactrian camel too, the average let down time is 58 seconds and it is not affected by massage of udder and teats for 20 seconds each and wiping the udder with damp cloth at 45°C or udder massage for 20 seconds and use of pre-heated teat cups of milking machine. However, milking time, milking rate and other milking traits (Table 45) may be affected by massage and heat treatment (Belokobylenko and Musaev, 1982). Machine milking in first calver bactrian heifers conditioned by twice daily udder massage for one and half months before calving significantly reduced let down time to only 18 seconds against 70 seconds for hand milked camels. Other milking traits are also affected (Musaev, 1982). The suckling, presence of the calf in front of dam and parentral administration of oxytocin have some effect on milking rate (Dynsembin, 1972)terminal phase of location (after 8-10 months) the camels (dromedary, bactrian and their Crossbreds) can be milked without calf (Blagovescenskii, 1963).

The camels are milked by both man and woman depending on the local traditions. The milker hangs the milk container with the help of a rope from his neck and milking is done in standing position. Normally lactating camels are docile and special restraining is not required for milking. However,in some animals require restrain and their hind limbs are fastened with a rope tied above hock joint in a figure of eight.

Table 45. Milking traits of camels.

Milking trais	Treatments before milking		
1. Effect of pre-treatments & teat massage, 20 see.	Normal Wiping of udder. Udder massage machine with damp cloth for 20 sec. & milking at 45°C & udder use of pre-heated cups.		
Let down time (sec.)	58	52	55
Milking time (min.)	6.2	4.3	5.0
Milking rate/min. (ml)	320	391	333
Hand stripped milk (ml)	72	62	97
Residual milk (ml)	199	213	149
Milk yie1d/milking (ml)	2254	1958	1913
Milking out percentage	88	86	92
2. Effect of udder massage during pregnancy in heifers			
	Hand milking		Machine milking
Let down time (sec.)	70		18
Milking time (min.)	4.5		3.2
Milking rate/min. (ml)	440		667
Hand stripped milk (ml)	0		22
Residual milk (ml)	280		187
Milk yield/milking (ml)	1670		2133
Milking out percentage	83.2		91.1
3. Effect of udder shape	Round udder		Gland defined udder
Milking time (min.)	4.0		4.0
Àv. milking rate/min. (ml)	592		393
Max. milking rate/min. (ml)	912		695
Milk yield/milking (ml)	2370		1570
4. Effect of calf	Calf suckled 3-4 sucks	Calf tied in front	Oxytocin inj. 5-10 IU i/m
Cistern milk (%)	4.1	4.4	3.4
Alveolar milk (%)	76.8	81.0	85.0
Stripped milk (%)	19.8	14.6	11.6

Variation in milking traits is quite high among the camels and these are influenced by mode of milking, massage of udder teats, milk production capacity, suckling by the calf and use of oxytocin (Dzhumagulov and Baimukanov, 1971) besides type, species, breed and lactation number, nutritional supply and dehydration.

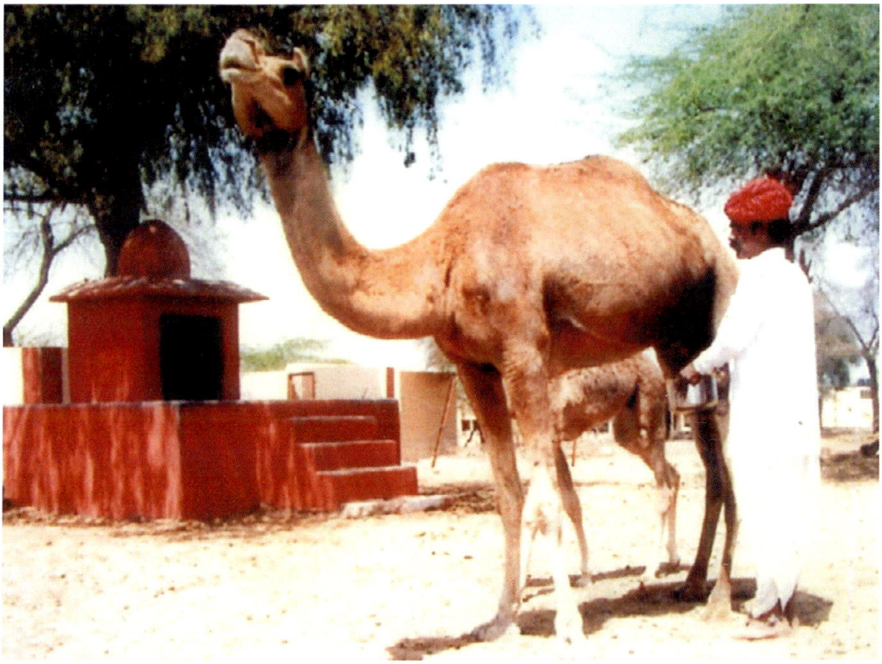

Milking

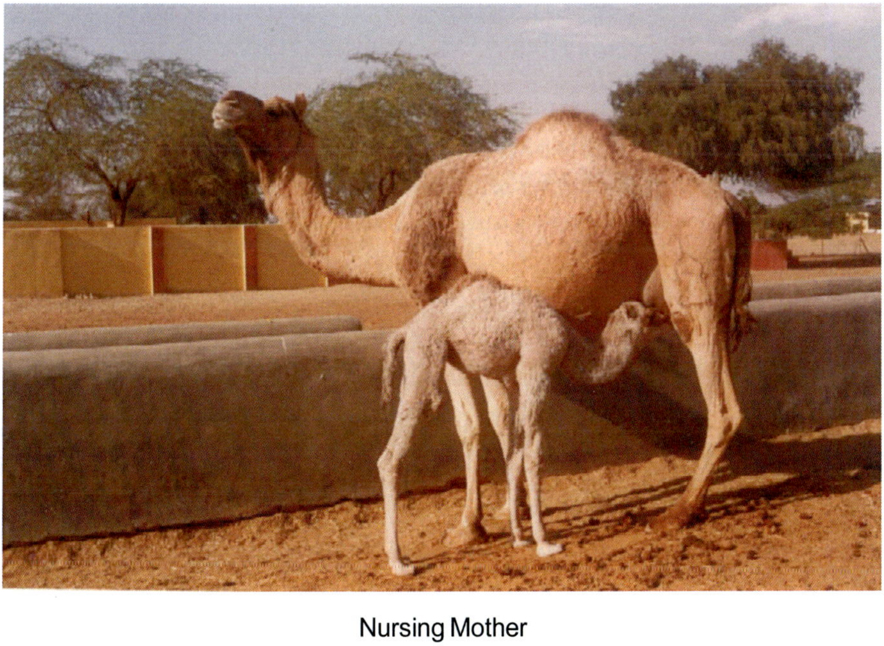

Nursing Mother

Milking frequency in camels

The camels are normally milked twice daily in most of the tropical countries both by the caleliars and also at the organised farms. The milking time is generally early morning and late in the evening. However, in Kenya thrice daily milking is done, i.e. once in daytime and twice in the night (Spencer, 1973). The milking frequency is generally irregular among the nomadics. The camels (dromedary, bactrian and their crossbreds) in cold desert of central Asia are usually milked three (Heraskov, 1965) or four times (Kulaeva, 1964) daily, and milking interval is about 8 and 6 hours respectively. While milking care is taken to spare sufficient milk in the udder for the suckling of the calf.

Colostrum

The first milk produced after the parturition is different in consistency and composition than the normal milk and it is called colostrum. Besides being highly nutritious, it also provides protection against many infectious diseases by supplying immuno-globulins (antibodies) which are not transmitted by the placenta in ruminants. This passive immunity provides protection in early life until the development of active immunity systems. The colostrum of camelids is yellowish white with slightly abnormal odour than the milk and unpleasant taste. Its consistency is thicker than the colostrum of cows and buffaloes due to higher viscosity, which is 1.72 times of water. Average values of specific gravity, refrective index, boiling point, titrable acidity after 12 h of milking and pH are 1.079, 1.382, 210°F (98.9°C), 0.38 per cent and 5.9 respectively, and clean milk is normally obtained after 4-6 days of calving (Ohri and Joshi, 1961a). The titrable: acidity in fresh colostrum is higher than the clean milk (0.2 vs 0.14 per cent) and it clots on heating (Khanna *et al.*, 1990).

There is a great difference in the composition of colostrum of Indian dromedary recorded by two groups (Ohri and Joshi,1961a and Khanna *et al.*, 1990). The values (Table 46) reported by the later group appears to be recorded after suckling by the calf for a day or two which is evident from almost similar values of total solids and lactose in colostrum and clean milk and this colostrum may be considered abnormal. The contents of total solids, protein, albumin, globulins and casein are also much higher in colostrum than the milk of bactrian camel without any significant difference in the values of ash, calcium and phosphorus (Dashdendev and Tretevich, 1964). The colostrum or dumber of camel is considered to possess laxative property and it is often used for drinking by the Somali people (Mares, 1954). In some parts of India, camel's colostrums spared from the suckling of calf is used for human consumption after coagulating by boiling. The whey is drained out and the clotted colostrum is after mixing sugar or jaggary.

Table 46. Percentage composition colostrum of Indian dromedary and bactrian camel.

Particulars	Water	TeS	SNF	Fat	Protein	Lactose	Ash
Maximum value*	78.7	27.8	27.4	0.4	19.5	5.1	2.8
Minimum value	72.2	21.3	21.2	0.1	15.8	4.0	1.4
Average value	75.2	24.8	24.6	0.2	17.7	4.3	2.6
Average value**	87.3	12.7	10.1	2.6	3.9	5.4	0.7
Bactrian***	69.6	30.4	30.2	0.2	19.4	7.2	3.6

*Ohri and Joshi (1961); **Khanna *et al.* (1990); ***Bestuzheva (1958).
T S = total solids; SNF = solids not fat.

The lack of transfer of immunoglobulins from the dam to foetus through placenta is evident from the non-detectable level of immunoglobulin IgG in the serum of newborn camel calf before suckling the colostrum from its dam. The mean value of IgG in the serum of she-camel on the day of parturition is about 33.09 + 5.5 mg per ml of serum. The content of IgG in pre-suckled colostrum ranges from 77 to 220 mg per ml on the day of parturition. The levels of IgG in the serum of colostrum had camel calves had been observed to be about 16, 12, 10 and 9-10 mg per ml at 7, 14, 21 and 28 days of age, respectively (Ungar-Waron it *et al.*, 1987). There is sudden increase in the IgG content of serum after the feeding of colostrum, which decreases sharply upto 21 days of age and thereafter, its level is more or less same upto 23 days of age.

The composition of colostrum changes rapidly following the suckling milking. The colostrum of bactrian camel contains 30.4% total solids, 0.2% fat, 19.4% protein, 7.2% lactose and 3.6% ash immediately after parturition and before suckling. With in 2 days of lactation, total solids reduces to 18.4% due to fall in protein to 3.6% (2.5% albumin + globulins and 1.1% casein) and in ash to 1.3%. However, fat increases to 5.8 % and lactose remains almost similar (Bestuzheva, 1968).

Milk of camelids

The whole milk of dromedary camel is an opaque white lacteal secretion obtained after about one week of calving. It is thicker than the cow milk and thinner than the buffalo milk. The odour is faintly sweetish and taste is sweet but sharp (Ohri and Joshi, 1961b). Normal milk of alpaca is also white in colour and slightly more sweet and viscous than the cow milk (Jimenez Ochoa, 1970). It is believed particularly in Arabia that the camel milk gives strength, virility and longivity (Sohail, 1983).

Physical properties of milk

The colour of clean milk is opaque white and odour is sweetish. It is viscous fluid slightly heavier than the water. Average viscosity of milk (27.8°C) is 1.17 times of water and the mean values of specific heat, refrective index and boiling point are 0.9465, 1.3495 and 212°F (98.8°C) respectively (Ohri and Joshi, 1961b). The freezing point depression of the milk of Egyptian dromedary is -0.576°C (E1-Bahay, 1962). The milk of bactrian camel is more or less similar to the dromedary milk (Cherepanova *et al.*, 1986a) while the milk of alpaca is more viscous (Jimenez Ochoa, 1970) The values of specific gravity of the milk of different species and types show considerable variation (Table 47).

Table 47. Specific gravity of milk of camelids.

Species/type	Specific gravity	Source
Milk of Dromedary,		
Egyptian	1.0305	El-Bahay, 1962
Egyptian	1.0320	Wahba *et al.*, 1988
Indian		1.0268 - 1.0356 Ohri & Joshi, 1961b
Milk of Bactrian	1.0290 – 1.0340	Kheraskov, P60
Milk of Alpaca	1.0265 – 1.0494	Jimenez Ochoa, 1980

The keeping quality of camel's milk is much longer than the woman's milk and bovine milk. Woman's milk becomes sour (pH 5.5 + 0.08) within 24 hours and cow's milk turns sour (pH 5.7 + 0.15) within 2 days, and both curdles at room temperature (30°C). However, camel's milk remains almost unchanged upto first 5 days and gradually becomes sour (pH 5.8 + 0.06) in next 2 days but does not coagulate for few months, when stored in sealed containers at room temperature (Yagil *et al.*, 1984). This may be due to high anti-bacterial activities and buffering ability in the camel's milk.

Anti-microbial properties of camel's milk

Reasonably high anti-microbial activities have been observed in the milk of bactrian (Kospakov, 1975) dromedary camels. Various protective proteins present in the milk of camels are lysozyme, lactoferrin, lactoperoxidase, immuno-globulins G and secretary immuno-globulin A. The lysozyme in camel milk has inhibitory action on Salmonella typhimurium and its activity is similar to yolk but it has no itic effect on Eschirichia coli and Staphyllococus aureus. The activity of lactoferrin is similar to that in cow milk and it inhibits S typhimurium (E1-Agamy *et al.*, 1992). Very little anti-bacterial activity has been observed in camel milk by whany lysozyme (Barbour *et al.*, 1984).

Composition of milk

There appears to be no standard for the composition of camel milk in the available literatures. There is considerable variation in the composition of milk of different camel species and also within the species (Table 48). The camel milk is slightly acidic with pH range 6.4 to 6.8 but it does not coagulate due to high buffering capacity.

Factors affecting the composition of camel's milk

The composition of milk is altered by several factors like species, type, location, farms, plane of nutrition and dehydration (Table 49). Milk composition specially the fat and protein contents are also affected by the month of lactation and lactational milk yield (Table 50).

The quality of milk changes drastically with the change in season. Dehydrated female camels secret highly diluted milk of low fat content. This physiological change is considered as superb adaptation for an arid environment. The calves are supplied sufficient water in addition to adequate supply of nutrients through diluted milk (Ahmed, 1990). Dehydration of lactating females results into greatest decrease in fat percentage followed by protein, lactose and ash contents (Yagil and Etzion, 1980).

Table 48. Percentage composition of milk and pH of milk of camelids

Species/type	Details	Water	T S	Fat	Protein	Lactose	Ash	pH	Reference
One-humped of Dromedary camel,									
Arabian		86.57	13.43	3.07	4.00	5.59	0.77		Sohail, 1983
Indian	Minimum	85.08	10.40	2.60	3.20	3.12	0.69		Ohri & Joshi, 1961b
	Maximum	89.60	14.92	5.50	5.30	6.41	1.40		
	Average	86.43	13.57	3.78	3.95	4.88	0.95	6.68	
Indian	88.50	11.5	2.2	2.8	5.6	0.69			Khanna *et al.*, 1990
Pakistan		87.26	12.74	2.6	3.23	6.26	0.65		Siddiqui & Bari, 1959
Egyptian		88.0	12.0	3.8	3.5	3.9	0.76	6.56	El-Bahay, 1962
Dromedary	Minimum	83.2	9.2	2.8	3.8	4.0	0.68		Abdel Rahim, 1987
	Maximum	89.7	15.4	3.6	4.4	5.2	0.76		
	Average	87.4	13.4	3.2	4.0	4.8	0.70		
Dromedary		88.51	11.49	3.45	3.00	4.17	0.82	6.53	Ahmed, 1990
Dromedary (Russian)		86.33	13.62	4.47	3.50	4.95	0.70		Heraskov, 1961
Two-humped or Bactrian camel,									
Russian		85.02	14.98	5.39	3.80	5.10	0.69		do
1	**2**	**3**	**4**	**5**	**6**	**7**	**8**	**9**	**10**
Central Asia		83.6	16.4	6.1	3.6	5.7	1.1		Bestuzheva, 1958
Russian	Minimum	85.12	12.66	4.47	3.2	4.3	0.69		Kheraskov, 1960
	Maximum	87.34	14.88	5.10	3.8	5.1	0.88		
Chinese	Minimum	82.8	13.0	4.0	3.7	3.2	0.95		Shirong & Shuzhen, 1984
	Maximum	87.0	17.2	7.6	4.1	5.2	0.98		
	Average	85.3	14.7	5.5	3.9	4.3	0.96		
New World Cameloids,									
Alpaca				4.4	5.67			6.6	Jimenez Ochoa, 1970
Llama		86.5	13.5	3.2	3.9	5.6	0.8		Altzan & Dittner, 1961

Table 49. Effect of species, location, farms, plane or nutrition and dehydration on milk composition.

Factor	TS	Fat	Protein	Lactose	Ash	Source
Species, types and location –						
Alpaca	-	4.4	5.7	-	-	Jimenez ochoa, 1970
Llama	13.5	3.2	3.9	5.6	0.8	Altman & Dittener, 1961
Bactrian camel -						
Chinese	14.7	5.5	3.9	4.3	0.96	Shirong & Shuzhen, 1984
Russian	15.0	5.4	3.8	5.1	0.7	Heraskov, 1961
Dromedary camel-						
Arabian	13.5	3.1	4.0	5.6	0.8	Sohail, 1983
Egyptian	12.0	3.8	3.5	3.9	0.8	El-Bahay, 1962
Indian	13.6	3.8	4.0	4.9	0.9	Ohri & Joshi, 1961b
Effect of farms-						
Farm I	14.38	4.96	4.13	4.65	0.64	Cherepanova *et al.*, 1986a
Farm II	14.27	4.77	4.21	4.61	0.68	
Effect of plane of nutrition –						
Good feeding	14.4	5.5	4.5	3.4	0.9	Knoess, 1977
Poor feeding	13.0	2.9	3.9	5.4	0.77	
Watered camels	14.3	4.3	4.6	4.6	0.6	Yagil & Etzion, 1980
Dehydrated camels	8.3	1.1	2.5	2.9	0.4	do

Table 50. Effect of lactation month and lactation milk yield on milk fat and milk protein in camels.

Factors		Milk fat	Milk protein	Source
Lactation month	5th	4.19	3.37	Cherepanova *et al.*,
	11th	5.91	4.51	1986b
Lactation milk				
yield (1)	300-500	5.10	4.36	
(Bactrian)	500-700	5.32	4.45	
	700-900	4.93	4.24	
	900-1100	5.08	4.15	
	1100-1300	4.74	3.85	
	1300-1500	4.10	3.65	
(Dromedary)	879	6.08		Kulaeva, 1964
	1205	6.59		
	1572	5.76		

Correlation between some milk constituents of bactrian camel

A significant correlation has been observed between fat and total solids (TS), protein and TS and fat and protein in the milk of Suni breed of two-humped camels of China (Shirong and Shuzhen, 1984). The values of correlation coefficients are as follows :

Correlation between milk fat vs TS - 0.89;

milk protein vs TS – 0.80; and

milk fat vs milk protein – 0.96

Proteins in camel milk

The larger portion of protein in milk is casein followed by lactalbumin and lactoglobulins. The later is maximum in colostrum which declines sharply. Fresh colostrum drawn just after parturition contains about 19.4 per cent protein formed of 18 per cent albumin and globulins and 1.4 per cent casein. After 2 days total protein fell down to 3.6 per cent containing 2.5 per cent albumin and globulins and 1.1 per cent casein (Bestuzheva, 1958). The ratio between casein and albumin is almost reversed in the clean milk and has been found to be more or less similar (Table 51) in the milk of bactrian and dromedary camels (Kheraskov, 1961) except an earlier report showed very low albumin content in the milk of dromedary of Pakistan (Siddiqui and Bari, 1959).

Table 51. Proteins in camel milk.

Species	Protein	Casein	Albumin	Whey protein	Source
Bactrian	4.32	3.2	0.15	-	Urbinsov *et al.*, 1981
Bactrian	3.8	2.9	0.97	-	Kheraskov, 1961
Dromedary	3.5	2.7	0.89	-	do
Dromedary	3.54	2.6	-	0.94	El-Bahay, 1962
Dromedary	3.23	3.11	0.12	-	Siddiqui & Bari, 1959

Various protective proteins in camel's milk are mostly enzymes like lysozyme, lactoferrin and lactoperoxidase, and immuno-globulins G and secretary immuno-globulin A (El-Agamy *et al.*, 1992).

The average content of alpha-lactalbumin in llama milk is least variable during the lactation period but highly variable between the animals. It has been reported to be 3.1 ± 0.74, 3.4 ± 0.34, 3.3 ± 0.97 and 3.8 ± 1.63 g/l in the milk of first, second, third to fifth and eight to tenth month of lactation respectively, with overall average 3.4 ± 0.97 g/l (Fernandez and Oliver, 1992). Amino acids in Camel milk in comparison to other ruminants and human milk.

The amino acids profile of the casein of dromedary milk has been compared with the milk of cow, goat and woman (Table 52). Variation in the amino acids content of casein of Sudanese camel is larger for aspartic acid, glutamic acid, leucine, proline and tyrosine. It also contained 1.72 ± 0.15 mg ammonia nitrogen per 100 g of casein (Hoeller and Hassan, 1965). The taurine content and free amino acids are much less in camel milk in comparison to goat milk and human milk. Non-protein nitrogen formed about 10.1, 7.8, 5.7 and 24.2 per cent of total protein in the milk of camel, goat, cow and woman respectively (Mehaia and Al-Kauhal, 1992).

Table 52. Amino acids profile of milk of some mammals.

Amino acids	*Bactrian	**Dromedary	**Goat	**Cow	Woman
Alanine	6.24	3.05 ± 0.20	3.55	3.41	3.5
Arginine	0.57	3.15 ± 0.26	2.10	4.14	3.17
Aspartic acid	10.12	7.65 ± 0.56	7.38	7.47	7.3
Glycine	5.14	1.57 ± 0.14	2.10	2.08	2.0
Glutamic acid	17.17	23.40 ± 0.78	20.32	23.16	23.4
Histidine	2.51	2.51 ± 0.20	4.99	3.02	2.6
Isoleudine	5.39	6.40 ± 0.28	4.31	6.60	6.4
Leucine	9.77	10.44 ± 0.52	9.94	10.00	9.8

Lysine	3.51	7.58 ± 0.28	8.23	8.06	7.8
Methionine	2.97	3.47 ± 0.19	3.54	3.19	2.5
Cysteine	-	-	-	-	0.9
Phenylalanine	2.98	5.64 ± 0.29	6.00	5.41	4.9
Proline	12.77	13.28 ± 0.82	14.59	11.83	11.1
Serine	6.81	5.88 ± 0.26	5.16	6.60	5.9
Threonine	6.47	6.31 ± 0.19	5.73	4.30	4.6
Tyrosine	2.55	5.76 ± 0.42	4.77	5.80	5.1
Valine	4.56	1.40 ± 0.35	5.69	7.47	6.9

* Urbimou *et al.*, 1981
** Hoeller and Hassan, 1965

Milk lipids

Lipids in camel milk is formed of 25.5 - 27.4, 26.6 -26.7, 11-11.7, 11.3-11.4, 10.8 and 3.1 per cent of oleic acid, palmitic acid, palmitoleic acid, myristic acid, stearic acid and linoleic acid respectively (Sawaya *et al.*, 1984; Ahmed, 1990). Camel milk contains more linoleic, linolenic and long chain polyunsaturated fatty acids than the cow milk and fat globule membrane contains about 35.5 per cent of the total phospholipids in the milk (Ahmed, 1990). Average size of fat globule of the milk is 2.9 μm and its number is about 5409 x 10^6 per ml (Wahba *et al.*, 1988).

The phospholipids composition of camel milk is by and large comparable with the milk of several mammalian species (Table 53) except that total choline phospholipids are less (Morrison, 1968).

Table 53. Distribution of phospholipids in mammalian milk.

Phospholipids	Camel	Cow	Buffalo	Ewe	Ass	Sow	Human
Phosphatidyl - ethanolamine	35.9	31.3	29.6	36.0	32.1	36.8	25.9
Phosphatidyl - choline	24.0	34.5	27.8	29.2	26.3	21.6	27.9
Phosphatidyl - serine	4.9	3.1	3.9	3.1	3.7	3.4	5.8
Phosphatidyl - inositol	5.9	4.7	4.2	3.4	3.8	3.3	4.2
Sphingomyelin	28.3	26.2	32.1	28.3	34.1	34.9	31.1
Lysophosphatidyl – ethanolamine	1.0	0.8	1.6	0.0	0.0	0.0	3.7
Lysophosphatidyl – choline	0.0	0.0	0.8	0.0	0.0	0.0	1.4
Total choline phospholipids	52.3	59.7	60.7	57.5	60.4	56.5	59.0

Minerals in milk

Various macro and micro minerals of nutrition significance observed in camel milk are calcium, phosphorus, magnesium, sodium, potassium, sulphur, copper, zinc and iron. The values of calcium and phosphorus in the milk of dromedary (Khan and Appanna, 1964; Wahba *et al.*, 1988) are comparable with the contents in the milk of Chinese bactrian camel (Shirong and Shuzhen, 1984) but the values of these elements in the milk of Russian bactrian camel (Cherepanova *et al.*, 1986) are almost double (Table 54).

Table 54. Minerals content in camel milk, mg/100 ml.

Species	Calcium	Magnesium	Phosphate	Source
Dromedary	109	9	127	Wahba *et al.*, 1988
do	128	18	97	Khan & Appanna,1964
Bactrian	100-110		80-100	Shirong & Shuzhen,
1984				
do	219		259	Cherepanova *et al.*,
do	217		270	1986 b

A comparison of minerals content in milk dry matter of single-humped camel and goat (Table 55) showed much lower concentration of most of the minerals in the milk of camel (Abdel-Rahim, 1987). Iron content in camel milk (0.32 mg/100 ml) is quite satisfactory to meet the nutritional requirements of the suckling calves (Khan and Appanna, 1964). Copper content (0.121-0.133 ppm) in dromedary milk is higher than 0.078-0.105 ppm in goat milk but lower than 0.2 - 0.232 ppm in cow milk and 0.192 - 0.218 ppm in buffalo milk (Baruah *et al.*, 1983).

Table 55. Minerals in the milk of camel and goat.

Minerals	Camel Milk	Goat Milk
Calcium (mg/g DM)	19.2 ± 2.9	30.2 ± 2.8
Phosphorus (mg/g DM)	7.4 ± 1.6	13.4 ± 1.8
Magnesium (mg/g DM)	0.69 ± 0.08	3.1 ± 0.58
Sodium (mg/g DM)	2.8 ± 0.22	2.4 ± 0.97
Potasium (mg/g DM)	12.3 ± 2.5	14.0 ± 2.7
Copper (mg/g DM)	6.5 ± 2.8	6.34 ± 2.1
Zinc (ug/g DM)	23.3 ± 6.7	55.3 ± 2.4
Iron (ug/g DM)	3.08 ±1.5	6.13 ± 0.68

Vitamins in camel milk

Only few information are available regarding carotenes and some vitamin in the milk of camel. The values of carotenes and vitamin A in the milk of dromedary are 9.41 (Range 5.2-12.46) and 7.57 (Range 4.84 -10.56) ug per ml respectively showed large variation between the animals (Khan and Appanna, 1965). In the milk of bactrian camel, vitamin A content is 0.037 mg and ascorbic acid is 5.7-9.8 mg per 100 ml (Kheraskov, 1960). Citrate content in the milk of Egyptian dromedary is about 148 mg per litre (Wahba *et al.*, 1988). Vitamin B12 and pantothenic acid content in the milk of bactrian camel (Table 56) are much less in comparison to most of the mammals (Kruglova and Bubnova, 1966).

Table 56. Some B vitamins in mammalian milk (per litre).

Species	Vitamin B_{12} (ug)	Biotin (ug)	Pantothenic acid (mg)
Antelope	2.9	72.2	5.1
Bactrian camel	1.7	-	0.6
Cow (Taurus)	4.4	47.7	4.3
Cow (Zebu)	2.8	58.5	3.0
Ewe	4.8	57.2	5.9
Goats	0.4	48.0	2.9
Mares	2.3	9.8	1.6

The differences in the concentration of B-vitamins may be due to difference in the types and number of rumen bacteria responsible for the synthesis of these vitamins.

Milk yield

Single-humped camels are generally good milkers and may continue to produce considerable amount of milk for more than 18 months when fodder supply is adequate and camels breeding is delayed. As high as 12,775 litres milk production in more than one year lactation in heavy camels of Pakistan (Morton, 1984) and upto 50 litres daily milk yield in some camels of northern Kenya (Field, 1980) has been reported. Average daily milk yield in Sakuye camels of northern Kenya is 4 litres, which is much higher than 0.5 litres daily milk of the local Kenyan cows (Yagil, 1986). The variation in milk production and lactation length of camels is very high and these are significantly influenced by several factors like species, type, breed, location, herbage cover, supplemental feeding, body weight and management, etc. (Rao, 1974, Morton, 1984, Richards and Gerard, 1985, Knoess *et al.*, 1986, Yagil, 1986, Khanna *et al.*, 1990). The milk production potential of double-humped camels is much less than the dromedaries under similar management (Dzhumagulov, 1983). Some information on milk yield, lactation length and other related traits of dromedary and bactrian camels have been summarized (Table 57). Inspite of the production ability of camels, they are not receiving proper treatment in many countries. A report from Turkman has shown gradual fall in the production of camels. The body weight of Turkman camel has drastically decreased from 500-600 kg in 1929 to 380-390 kg in 1982 and it has also adversely affected the production potential (Bairamov and Guvrichkin, 1983).

The small size South American cameloids are normally not milked and allowed nursing their cria for several months. The small quantity of milk spared from suckling of cria is milked for human consumption from alpaca. There is great variation in the quantity of spared milk and it ranges from as little as 40 ml to as high as 1200 ml per day (average 218 ml per day) in Peru (Jimenez ochoa, 1970).

Table 57. Milk yield and milk production traits of camels of different countries.

Species/location	Body wt. (kg)	Milk yield (1 or kg) Daily	Lactation	% of bwt.	305 days	Lactation length (month)	Source
1	2	3	4	5	6	7	8
Dromedary (Camelus dromedarius)							
Algeria	-	4.0-10.0	-	-	-	-	Gast *et al.*, 1969
Arabia	-		2000-3000	-	-	16-17	Sohail, 1983
China		7.5	-	-	-	16-17	Ensminger & Ensminger, 1973
Egypt	-	3.5 – 4.5	1600-2000	-	1078-1373	-	El-Bahay, 1962
	-	10.0-15.0	3000-4000	-	-	-	Shalash, 1979
Ethiopia	409	7.6	2774	1.86	-	12	Knoess, 1977
	360	5.0-13.0	1872-2592	1.4-3.6	1525-3965	12-18	Morton, 1984
(Dankali)	-	-	1123	-	-	12.25	Richards & Gerard, 1985
India (Bikaneri)	-	1.8-4.5	-	-	-	7-18	Sharma & Bhargava, 1963
	-	6.0-15.0	2000-3000	-	-	12	Rao *et al.*, 1970
	-	4.5-18.2	2430-8190	-	1373-5551	15-18	Rao, 1974
	-	3.8-10.8	-	-	-	9-18	Khanna *et al.*, 1990
Israel	-	7.0-15.0	-	-	-	9-18	Yagil & Etzion, 1980
1	2	3	4	5	6	7	8
Kenya	550	2.8-17.0	-	-	-	-	Field, 1979
Libya	380-400	8.3-10.0	2700-4000	2.2 – 2.6	2532-3050	9-16	Morton, 1984
Pakistan	-	9.1-13.6	2721-3629	-	-	16-18	Yasin & Wahid, 1957

	-	4.0-20.0	1000-5000	1.3-4.0	-	9-18	Knoess, 1982
(Heavy)	450	15.0-35.0	5475-12775	3.3-7.8	4515-10675	12	Morton, 1984
(Desert)	350	8.0-10.0	2920-3650	2.3-2.9	2440-3050	12	
Somalia	350	5.0	1950	1.4	1525	13	Morton, 1984
Sudan	-	5.0-10.0	1200-2600	-	-	10-12	El-Amin,1979
Russia	-	-	2000	-	-	7	Dzhumagulov, 1983
Tunisia	-	4.0	1220	-	1220	12	Burgemeister, 1974
Turkman	-	12.4	2000-3000	-	-	-	Bairamov & Gavrichlin, 1983
	900	-	1500-1700	-	-	7	Meredov, 1984
Bactrian (Camelus bactrianus)							
Astarkhan	450-500	-	1500	-	-	16-18	Teretjev, 1963
Kazakh & Kalmyk	-	-	879-1572	-	-	-	Kulaeva, 1964
Kazak	-	6.0-7.0	850	-	-	-	Aueljbekov, 1967
	-	4.8	868	-	-	6	Baimkuanov, 1969
Turkman	-	3.1-4.2	1500-2000	-	-	16-18	Diusembin, 1972

Effect of season on milk yield

Significant effect of season on milk yield is observed in both bactrian and dromedary camels. The season has conspicuous effect on the quantity and feeding value of herbages on the natural pastures which are ultimately responsible for the supply of nutrients for supporting production. Average daily milk yield of bactrian camel is 1.1 kg in winter and it is less than one-fourth of 4.84 kg daily milk yield in summer of central Asia (Be1okobylenko and Musaev, 1982).

Effect of feed availability on milk yield

The herbage cover and levels of nutrients supply are apparently reflected in milk yield and lactation length (Table 58).

Table 58. Effect of feeding levels on milk production.

Type of feed/level of feeding	Lactation length (days)	Milk yield (1/kg.)	Source
Bactrian camel			
Poor feeding	-	1.10/day	Belokobylenko &
Good feeding	-	4.84/day	Musaev,1982.
Dromedary camel			
Central Asia			
Poor feeding	540	1700/lact.	Iwema, 1960
Good feeding	540	upto 3000/lact.	
India			
Desert grazing	540	2430-4914/lact.	Rao, 1974
Irrigated fodder	450	3105-8190/1act.	
Pakistan			
Rainfed fodder	540	1506/lact.	Khan Sial, 1950
Irrigated fodder	540	2823/lact.	
Pakistan (Punjab)			
Poor feeding	270-540	1350/lact.	Knoess, 1977
Good feeding	270-540	2700-3600/lact.	

Effect of water restriction on milk yield

An increase in in milk though containing much less solids and high water content has been observed in dromedaries due to restricted water supply for drinking causing partial dehydration (Table 59). The water content in normal milk of hydrated camel is about 85 per cent which increased to more than 90 per cent due to drastic reduction in fat content on restricting water intake. Water restriction also causes considerable drop in protein, lactose an mineral contents of milk (Yagil and Etzion, 1980). Lactating animals secret large volume of water in milk. The milk secretion is controlled by coordinated action of anti-diuretic hormone (ADH) and aldosterone alongwith the normal hormones prolactin and oxytocin responsible for the secretion and let down of milk. Besides ADH, oxytocin and prolactin are also anti-diuretic in action and help in water supply for secretion in milk and this action increases in camels on dehydration as suggested by Yagil and Etzion (1980). The role of ADH and aldosterone, in the maintenance of milk production and secretion of highly diluted milk received support from the results of experiment on laboratory mammals (Etzion and Yagil, 1981).

Table 59. Effect of water restriction on milk yield.

Season	Watering	Milk yield/day(l)
Early sprin	Ad libitum	3.7 ± 0.2
Late spring	Restricted	5.7 ± 0.4
Early summer	Restricted	6.0 ± 0.3
Mid summer	Restricted	6.2 ± 0.4
Late summer	Restricted	6.0 ± 0.5

Effect of body weight (probably breed) on milk production

The heavy camels of Pakistan described as plain type produce much higher quantity of milk than the light weight camels of Pakistan described as desert type (Table 60) in about one year lactation (Morton, 1984).

Table 60. Effect of body weight on milk production.

Milk production traits	Heavy type	Light type
Type of camel	Plain type	Desert type
Body weight (kg)	450	350
Milk yield/day (kg)	15-35	8-10
Milk yield/lactation (kg)	5475-12775	2920-3650
Milk yield as % of bwt.	3.3-7.8	2.3-2.9
Milk yield adjusted for 365 days (kg)	4575-10675	2440-3050
Lactation length (month)	12	12

Effect of hybridization on milk production

An increase in milk production has been observed in crossbred camels (Bactrian X Dromedary and Dromedary X Bactrian) and inter-species crossbreeding is quite popular in central Asia and China for increased production. About 25 to 40-50 per cent increase in milk production has been reported in the hybrids (Blagovascenskii, 1963, Belokobylenko, 1982 and Dzhumagulov, 1983). A comparision of milk production in pure bred and hybrid camels (Table 61) has been made in some studies (Baimukanov, 1969 and Dzhumagulov, 1983).

Table 61. Milk production in pure bred and hybrid camels.

Type of camel	Milk yield (kg)			Source
	Daily	Lactation		
Kazakh bactrian (KB)	4.8	868	6	Baimukanov, 1969
KB x Dromed cross	5.3-12.7	962-2277	6	
Bactrian		1180	7	Dzhumagulov, 1983
Dromedary		2000	7	
Bact X Drom & reciprocal		1980	7	

Comparison of milk production traits of camel with common dairy animals

It is well known that in dry areas camels thrive better than most of the ruminant species. A comparative study on camles (Camelus dromedarius), buffaloes (Bubalus bubalis), Sahiwal cows of zebu cattle (Bos indicus) and Frisien X Sahiwal (Bos Taurus X Bos indicus) crossbred cows (Table 62) under identical agro-climatic conditions of the Punjab province of Pakistan shows that plain type camels of Pakistan produce much higher milk in comparison to even dairy type cattle (Knoess *et al.*, 1986).

Tab1e 62. Comparison of milk production of dairy animals.

Species	Number of animals	Body weight (kg)	Milk yield kg/day	Milk yield %of bwt.	Fat in milk (%)
Camel	5	574	18.68	3.26	2.93
Buffalo	14	630	6.80	1.08	5.59
Sahiwal cow	14	400	11.10	2.78	4.47
Frinsien X Sahiwal cross	14	400	11.97	2.99	4.17

Milk Products

Different kinds of milk products are prepared from the camel milk. As usual common milk products prepared in Indian subcontinent are khoa (evaporated whole milk, butter, ghee (clarified milk fat) and sweats prepared from khoa (Aggarwala and Sharma, 1961, Rao *et al.*, 1970, Knoess *et al.*, 1986). Butter is also prepared in Egypt (Shalash, 1980) and neighbouring countries. In addition to butter, aaruul a hard, dry and cubed cheese, soft cheese, fermented milk products and distillates are prepared in Mongolia (Namekh and Accolas, 1978, Chapman, 1985) and similar products in China (Dong Wei, 1980). Fermented coumis like milk products are more common in central Asia like subert in the Kazakhastan, cal or chal in the Turkman and azran in the Uzbekistan (Heraskov, 1961, 1965).

Cream, butter and ghee

Separation of fat in the form of cream and butter is somewhat tidious in comparison to cow and buffalo milk due to smaller size of fat globules in camel's milk. The size of fat globules in camel milk ranges from 2.00 to 3.93 um (Wahwa *et al.*, 1983, Gouda *et al.*, 1984, Knoess *et al.*, 1986, Farah and Ruegg, 1991). Natural cream separation from camel milk is very poor (Farah and Ruegg, 1991) and it requires 5-6 days refrigeration for satisfactory cream separation (Abu-Lehia, 1989). Satisfactory cream seperation has been reported on centrifugation of boiled milk at 33.7-45°C (Knoess *et al.*, 1986, Hagrass *et al.*, 1987, Abu-Lehia *et al.*, 1989).

Butter is prepared from boiled milk after souring and churning (Knoess *et al.*, 1986). Butter from sweet cream may be prepared by traditional churning (Hagrass *et al.*, 1987) and higher butter fat yield may be obtained by hand churning of sweet cream at 25°C (Farah *et al.*, 1989). However, churning of sour cream is more easy and faster but losses are higher. The butter made of camel milk is white, waxy, sticky and greasy (Farah *et al.*, 1989).

Ghee is prepared from butter by usual boiling at low heat for the separation of fat after evaporation of moisture and precipitation of proteinous fraction (Aggarwala and Sharma, 1961).

Khoa making

Khoa is prepared by evaporation of moisture to the extent of about 80 per cent on low heat. The boiling milk is continuously stirred with a wooden ladle during the process of khoa making.

Cheese making

Coagulation of camel milk by rennet is difficult and even the use of additives like calcium chloride, calcium phosphate, higher amount of rennet and changing of pH and temperature could not produce satisfactory effect on clotting time (Ramet, 1987, Farah and Bachmann, 1987, Mohamed *et al.*, 1989, Bayoumi, 1990). In most of the cases, the milk generally flocculates which makes cheese making difficult. However, in many countries processes of cheese making have been developed and it is quite common in central Asian countries. A very granular, friable and white cheese is prepared from the naturally soured milk (Purchase, 1943). A hard cheese is prepared by adding whey culture in the milk (Mohamed *et al.*, 1990). Addition of whey culture increases the hardness of the coagulum and reduces clotting time but in this process also about half of the milk fat is retained in the whey (Kamoun and Bergaoui, 1989).

Fermented milk products

Fermented milk beverages like chal and shubat resembling koumiss are commonly prepared in the central Asian countries. Methods for the commercial preparation of chal and kefir have been briefly described (Rao *et al.*, 1970). For the manufacture of kefir, the milk is flash pasteurized at 85°C, cooled to 26-30°C, inoculated with kefir culture (3-6 %) and bottled. During the process of incubation for 8-12 hours at 20-26°C, a soft coagulum is formed. The product is now ripened at 6-8°C for 24-28 hours. The product, kefir has refreshing flavour, thick creamy texture, white appearance and also contains gas. Chal is also a white and sour beverage. It is prepared by using the cultures of Lactobacillus casei, Streptococcus thermophilus and lactose fermenting yeasts, by incubating a 25°C for 8 hours and then at 20°C for 16 hours. In Iran, chal is manufactured from unheated camel milk subjected to both acid and alcohol fermentation (Karim and Taghdisian, 1990).

References

Abdul Rahim, A.G. 1987. The chemical composition and nutritional value of camel (Camelus dromaderius) and goat (Capra hircus) milk. World Rev. anim. Prod., 23:9.

Abu-Lehia, I.H., Al-mohizea, I.S. and El-behry, M. 1989. Studies on the production of ice-cream from camel milk products. Australian J. Dairy Technol., 44:31.

Aggarwala, A.C. and Sharma, 1961.

Ahmed, M.M. 1990. The analysis and quality of camel's milk. Thesis, University of Reading, U.K.

Altman, P.L. and Dittmer, D.S. (Eds.) 1961. Blood and other body fluids. Fed. American Soc. Exp. Biol., Washington.

Aueljbekov, K. 1967. Camel breeding – a profitable field. Konevod. Konnyi Sport, 5:6.

Bairamov, D. and Gavrichkin, v. 1983. Camels should be returned to the desert. Konevo. Konnyi Sport, 7:11.

Baruah, S., Garg, B.S., Singh, R.P. and Singh, I. 1983. A rapid spectrophotometric method for trace determination of copper in milk. J. Indian Chem. Sec., 60:64.

Bayoumi, S. 1990. Studies on composition and rennet coagulation of camel milk. Milchwirtschachaf. Forschung., 42:3.

Belokobylenko, V.T. 1982. Zootechnical background to the production of shubat at modern farms. Dairy Sc., Abstr., (1984), 46:652.

Belokobylenko, V.T. and Musaev, Z.M. 1982. Machine milking of camels without suckled calved. Dairy Sci. Abstr, 46:652.

Bestuzheva, K.T. 1958. Composition of the colostrum and milk of camel. Dairy Sci. Abstr., 20:1039.

Blagovescenskii, V. 1963. Reserves in the production of milk and meat. Konevod. Konnyi Sport, 33:8.

Burgemeister, R. 1975. Elevage de chameaux en Afrique du Mord. 86 pp. GZT, Eschborn.

Charpman, M.J. 1985. Mongolia: bactrian camels. World Anim. Rev. No. 55:14.

Cherepanova, V.P. and Belokobylenko, V.T. 1986. The correlation between fat and protein in the milk of camels. Zhivotnovo-dstvo No. 10:33.

Cherepanova, V.P., Musaev, Z.M. and Belokobylenko, V.T. 1986. The chemical composition of camel milk. Zhivotnovodstvo No. 3:55.

Dashdendev, D. and Tretevich, V.I. 1964. The chemical composition of chamel's milk. Resp. nauch. Konf. po Fiziol. Biokhim. Sel khoz. Zhivot., Lvov. Sb. P. 85.

Cossins, N.J. 1971. Pastoralism under pressure. Report, Livestock meat board, Addis Abeba.

Dynsembin, Kh. 1972. Milk ejection in the female camel. Trudy institute Fiziologii, Alma-Ata, Kazakhastan, 17:33.

Dzhumagulov, I.K. 1983. Hybridization in camel breeding. Zhivotnovodstvo No. 9:46.

Dzhumagulov, I.K. and Baimukanov, A.B. 1971. Physiological characters of lactation and milking rate in the camel. Vest. Sel'-khoz. Nauki, Alma-Ata, 14(9):46.

El-Agamy, E.I., Ruppanner, R., Ismail, A., Champagne, C.P. and Assaf, R. 1992. Anti-bactrial and anti-viral activity of camel milk protective protein. J. Dairy Res., 59:169.

El-Amin, F.M. 1979. the dromedary camel of Sudan. Proc. IFS Intern. Symposium, Sudan, p. 35.

El-Bahay, G.M. 1962. Normal contents of Egyptian camel milk. Vet. Med. J., 8:7.

Ensminger, M.S. and Ensminger, A. 1973. China: the impossible dream. Agricultural Service Foundation, Clovis.

Etzion, Z. and Yagil, R. 1981. Effect of exogenous ADH and aldosterone on milk in heat-stressed animals. Comp. Biochem. Physiol. 69A: 129.

Farah, Z. and Bachmann, M.R. 1987. rennet coagulation properties of camel milk. Milchwiss., 42:689.

Farah, Z. and Ruegg, M.W. 1991. The creaming properties and size distribution of fat globules in camel milk. J. Dairy Sci., 74:2901.

Farah, Z., Streif, T. and Bachmann, M.R. 1989. Manufacture and characteristics of camel milk butter. Milchwiss., 44:412.

Fernandez-baca, S. 1975. alpaca raising in the high Andes. World Animal Review No. 14:1.

Fernandez, F.M. and Oliver, G. 1992. Studies of alpha-lactoalbumin in llama milk. Small Rumin-Res., 8:07.

Field, C.R. 1980. Camel growth and milk production in Marsabit district, North Kenya. Prov. Report, Intern. Foundation of Science No. 6:215.

Gast, M., Maubois, J.L., and Adda, J. 1969. Le lait et les products laitiers on a Haggar. Centr. Rech. Anthrop., Prehist. Ethn.

Gouda, A., El-Zayat, A. and El-Shabarawy, S.A. 1984. Electron microscopy study on the size distribution of casein micelles, fat globules and fat globule membrane of camel milk. Annals Agric. Sci., Ain Shams Uni., 20:755.

Hagrass, A.E., Hassan, A.A., Soryal, K.A., Mervat, A.S. and El-Shabrawy, S.A. 1987. Chemical composition of fat and butter of camel's milk. Egyptian J. Food Sci., 15:15.

Heraskov, S.G. 1953. Camel's milk and its products. Konevod. Konnyi Sport, 23(11):35.

Hereskov, S.G. 1965. Camel milk: A valuable food product. Konevod. Konnyi Sport, 35(8):14.

Hoeller, H. and Hassan, Y.M. 1965. the amino acid compositon of camel milk casein, Sudan J. Vet. Sci., 6:60.

Iwema, S. 1960. The ship of the desert. Veeteelt-en Zuivelberichten, 3:390.

Jimenez ochoa, R. 1970. Some aspects of alpaca milk. Tropicales y de Altura, Peru No. 4:60.

Kamoun, M. And bergaoui, R. 1989. Un essai de production et transformation de lait de dromedaire en Tunisie. Revista Elev. Med. Vet. Pays Trop., 42:113.

Karim, G. and Taghdissian, H. 1990. "Chal" A fermented camel's milk. IDF Congress, Montreal, Canada.

Khan, M.K.U. and Appanna, T.C. 1965. Evaluation of biological value of camel milk protein. Indian J. Nutr. Dietet., 2:109.

Khanna, N.D., Tandon, S.N. and Rai, A.K. 1990. Breeding parameters of Indian camels. Indian J. Anim. Sci., 60:1347.

Kheraskov, S.G. 1960. Camel's milk as human food. Dairy Sci. Abstr., (1963), 25:250.

Knoess, K.H. 1977. The camel as a meat and milk animal. World Animal Review No. 22:39.

Knoess, K.H., Makhudum, A.J., Rafiq, M. and Hafeez, M. 1986. Milk production potential of dromedary with special reference to the province of Punjab, Pakistan. World Animal Review No. 57:11.

Kaspakov, Zh. K 1975. Antibactrial properties of camel's milk. Trudy Vsesoy. Nauchini-issled. Inst. Vet. Sanitarri, 51:37.

Kruglova, L.A. and Bubnova, V.P. 1966. Contents of vitamin B12, biotin and pantothenic acid in the milk of various animals. Dokl. Mosk. Sel'khoz. Akad. Timiryazeva, 127:105.

Kulaeva, V. 1964. The production of bactrian milk. Konevod. Konnyi Sport, 34:9.

Mares, R.G. 1954. Animal husbandry, animal industry and animal diseases in the Somaliland protectorate. British Vet. J., 110:411.

Mehaia, M.A. and Al-Kauhal, M.A. 1992. Taurine and other free amino acids in milk of camel, goat, cow and man. Milchwiss., 47:351.

Meredov, B. 1984. Some problems of camel breeding in Turkmenia. Konevod. Konnyi Sport. No, 12:22.

Mohamed, M.A., Larsson-Raznikiewicz, M. and Mohamed, M.A. 1990. hard cheese making from camel milk. Milchwiss., 45:716.

Mohamed, M.A., Mursal, A.I. and Larsson-Raznikiewicz, M. 1989. Separation of camel milk casein fraction and its relation to coagulation properties of milk. Milchwiss., 44:278.

Morrison, W.R. 1968. The distribution of phospholipids in some mammalian milks. Lipids, 3:101.

Morton, R.H. 1984. Camels for meat and milk production in Sub-Sahara Africa. J. Dairy Sci., 67:1548.

Musaev, Z.M. 1982. Milk production of Kazakh bactrian camel at mechanized farms. Dairy Sci. Asbtr., 46:5736.

Mosier, M.B. 1973. Histological structure of the mammary glands of the one humped camel (Camelus dromaderius). Indian J. Anim. Sci., 43:639.

Ohri, S.P. and Joshi, B.K. 1961a. Composition of colostrums of camel. Indian vet. J., 38:604.

Ohri, S.P. and Joshi, B.K. 1961b. Composition of milk of camel. Indian vet. J., 38:514.

Osman, D.I. and Ismail, H.I. 1988. Morphology of the camel udder. Arts working paper-camel forum No. 29:22 (Dairy Sci. Abstr., 1991, 53:117.

Pathak, N.N. 1990. Feeding standard of buffalo. Indian Veterinary Research Institute, Izatnagar, 243 122, India.

Purchase, H.S. 1943. Some experiments in the making of butter, ghee and cheese from camel's milk. East Afric. Agric. J., 9:38.

Ramet, J.P. 1987. Use of bovine calf rennet to coagulate raw camel milk. World Animal Review No. 61:11.

Ramet, J.P. 1989. L' aptitude from agere du lai de dromadaire. Revista Elev. Med. Vet. Pays Trop., 42:105.

Rao, C.K. 1974. Scheme for the improvement of Indian camels. Mmeo Item 7 and 10, Ministry of Agric., New Delhi.

Rao, M.B., Gupta, R.C. and Dastur, N.N. 1970. Camel's milk and milk products. Indian J. Dairy Sci., 23:71.

Richards, D. and Gerard, D. 1985. Milk production in Dankali dromedaries (Ethiopia). Proc. Intern. Congress Anim. Prod., Damascus, Syria.

Saleh, M.S., Mobarak, A.M. and Fouad, S.M. 1971. Radiological, anatomical and histological studies on the mammary gland of the one humped camel (Camelus dromaderius). 1. The teat. Zbl. Vet. Med. (A) 18:347.

Sawaya, W.N., Khalil, J.K., Al-Shalhat, A. and Mohammed, H. 1984. Chemical composition and nutritional quality of camel milk. J. Food Sci., 49:744.

Shalash, M.R. 1979. Utilization of camel meat and milk in human nourishment. Proc. IFS Intern. Symp. Camels, Sudan, p. 285.

Sharoha, A.M. 1987. Effect of the presence of calf and early weaning on milk secretion and growth rate of the young dromedary camel. Proc. Intern. Conf. Anim. Prod. in Arid zonas (ICPZ), Damascus, Syria.

Sharma, V.D. and Bhargava, K.K. 1963. The Bikaneri camel. Indian vet. J., 40:639.

Shirong, Shui and Shuzhen, Xu. 1984. Preliminary analysis of the quality of milk from the special Suni two-humped camel. Chinese J. Anim. Sci., 2:11.

Siddiqui, R.H. and Bari, M.A. 1959. Examination of milk and fat of camel. Chemical Abstract, 53:18322C.

Sohail, M.A. 1983. The role of the Arabian camel (Camelus dromaderius) in animal production. World Rev. Anim. Prod., 19:37.

Spencer, P. 1973. Nomads in alliance: symbiosis and growth among the Rendille and Samburu of Kenya, 230 pp. Oxford University Press, London.

Terentjev, S.M. 1963. Camel breeding in Astrakhan. Zivotn., 25:54.

Ungar-Waron, H., Elias, E., Cluckman, A. and Trainin, Z. 1987. Dromedary IgG: Purification, characterization and quantitation in sera of dams and newborns. Israel J. Vet. Med., 43:198.

Urbinsov, Zh.K., Servetnik-Chalaya, G.K. and Izatullaev, E.A. 1981. Protein composition of camel's milk. Vopr. Pitan., 6:41.

Wahba. A., El-Abbassy, F., Ismail, I. and El-Agamy, S.I. 1988. Studies on some physical properties of camel's milk. Egyptian J. Dairy Sci., 16:19.

Yagil, R. 1986. The camel self-sufficiency in animal protein in drought-stricken areas. World Animal Review, 57:2.

Yagil, R. and Etzion, Z. 1980. Milk yield of camel (Camelus dromaderius) in drough areas. Comp. Biochem. Physiol., 67A:207.

Yagil, R. and Etzion, Z 1980a. Effect of drought condition on the quality of camel milk. J. Dairy Res., 47:159.

Yagil, R., Saran, A. and Etzion, Z. 1984. Camel's milk: for drinking only? Comp. Biochem. Physiol., 78A:263.

❑❑❑

Chapter 6

Growth in Camelids

Growth is an important measure of production potential of farm animals and it is influenced by several factors like heredity, environment and management.

Body Weight at Birth or Birth Weight

The body weight at birth ranges from 25 to 52 kg in different kinds of bactrian and dromedary camel (Bhargava *et al.*, 1965, Burgemeister, 1975, Dong Wei, 1979) and 5.7 to 10 kg in various llamoid species (Rodriguez and Torres-Hernandez, 1982, Vorano and Bertoni, 1984). The birth weight is influenced by several factors like species, breed, location, sex of the calf, parity, month of calving, body weight of the dam and sire, etc.

1. Effect of species on birth weight

The average body weight of calves of different camel species and crias of the various cameloid species shows great variation (Table 63). Average birth weight of the large sized Indian dromedary is generally higher than the dromedary of Sudan and bactrian camels. Similarly, the birth weight of llama is higher than the birth weight of alpaca. The vicuna is the smallest camelid.

Table 63. Effect of species on birth weight.

Species	Birth weight (kg)	Source
Bactrian	35.0	Chapman, 1985
Dromedary, Indian	42.5	Beniwal & Chawdhry, 1983
Dromedary Sudan	32.5	Degan *et al.*, 1987
Alpaca	8.0	Fernandez-Baca, 1975
Llama	9.7	Rodriguez & Torres-Hernandez, 1982

2. Effect of breed on birth weight

Average birth weight of Bikaneri camels is generally higher than most of the other Indian breeds similar agro-climatic conditions and management. There is some contradiction in the mean birth weight of the Kutchi and Jaisalmeri breeds reared on the organised farms (Table 64).

Table 64. Effect of breed on birth weight.

Breed of dromedary	Birth weight (Kg.)	Source
Bikaneri	40.45 ± 0.64	Khanna *et al.*, 1990
Kutchi	34.00 ± 1.09	
Jaiselmeri	28.78 ± 1.20	
Arab X Bikaner	37.50 ± 1.25	
Bikaneri	33.75 ± 2.00	Anonymous, 1992-93
Kutchi	30.25 ± 1.67	
Jaiselmeri	31.22 ± 1.66	
Arab X Bikaneri	26.00 ± 2.00	

3. Effect of location on birth weight

The birth weight of Russian (Central Asian) and Mongolian bactrian is generally higher than the Chinese bactrian. Similarly, the birth weight of Indian dromedary is higher than the Sudanese and Tunisean dromedary (Table 65).

Table 65. Effect of location on birth weight.

Species	Location	Birth Wt. (Kg.)	Source
Bactrian	Russia	35-40	Aueljbekov, 1967
	Mongolia	35.4	Pansenko & Luvsan, 1971
	China	33.3	Dong Wei, 1979
Dromedary	India	42.5	Beniwal & Chowdhry, 1983
	Sudan	32.5	Degan *et al.*, 1987
	Kenya	30.9	Burgemeister, 1975
	Tunisia	25.2	

4. Effect of hybridization and crossbreeding on birth weight.

Two reports on the birth weight of Arab X Bikaneri camels are contradictory (Khanna *et al.*, 1990, Anonymous, 1992-93). The dromedary of the semi-desert of Kazakhstan is lighter in body weight than the bactrian camels of the region but yield more milk due to which hybrid breeding between dromedary and bactrian is quite popular as the hybrids are larger, produce more milk and meat and also work more. The hybrids produce about 20, 25 and 10 per cent more body weight, milk and wool respectively than the mid-parents production (Dzhumagulov, 1983). The crossbreds between the Astarkhan X Kazakh breeds mature earlier. They are more viable and yield more fibre (Terentjev, 1951).

5. Effect of the sex of calf on birth weight

Average birth weight of male calves is generally higher than the female calves in almost all kinds of camels and cameloids (Table 66). However, contradictory mean birth weights have been reported in observations on Bikaneri camels (Barhat *et al.*, 1979, Barhat and Chowdhary, 1980), which may be due to large difference in the number of observations or the ratio of male and female calves in the two studies.

Table 66. Effect of the sex of calves on birth weight.

Sex of calf/Species	Birth wt. (kg)	Source
Bactrian male, China	34.9	Dong Wei, 1979
do female	31.7	
do male, Mongolia	35.9	Panasenko & Luvsan,1971
do femle	34.8	
Bikaneri male, India	38.2	Bhargava *et al.*, 1965
do female	37.2	
do male	42.6	Barhat & Chowdhary, 1980
do female	40.6	
do male	44.3	Barhat *et al.*, 1979
do female	44.4	

6. Effect of parity on birth weight

Average birth weight of the calves of first calvers is normally lowest and it increases gradually with the subsequent calvings (Table 67). Such increase in birth weight has been so far observed upto third parity in Bikaneri camels (Bhargava *et al.*, 1965) and in the first and second parity of llamas (Vorano and Bertoni, 1984).

Table 67. Effect of parity on birth weight.

Parity	Birth weight (kg)	Source
Dromedary (Bikaneri)		
First	37.25 ± 0.43	Bhargava *et al.*, 1965
Second	38.47 ± 0.73	
Third	39.23 ± 1.64	
Llama		Vorano & Bertoni, 1984
First	6.15 (5.7-6.9)	
Second	8.37 (8.0-8.6)	

7. Effect of calving month on birth weight.

Average birth weight of Bikaneri camels has been found to be maximum for the January or December born calves and minimum for the May born calves (Table 68). Least variation has been observed in the birth weight of calves born from January to April in most of the observations.

Table 68. Effect of calving month on birth weight.

Month of calving	Birth weight Record 1	(Kg) Record 2	Record 3
December	41.54	42.86 ± 0.93	46.43 ± 0.85
January	37.39	41.38 ± 0.55	50.99 ± 0.88
February	37.49	41.02 ± 0.53	40.06 ± 0.85
March	38.22	41.02 ± 0.68	40.00 ± 0.86
April	38.42	-	-
May	36.68	-	-

Record 1, Bhargawa *et al.*, 1965; 1, Barhat & Chowdhary, 1980; 3, Barhat *et al.*, 1979.

8. Effect of the body weight of dams on birth weight.

The body weight of dam before calving has significant effect on birth weight of the calves (Table 69). Average birth weight of the calves of light size females is lowest and it increases with the corresponding increase in the body weight of dams. However, there is considerable difference in the observations recorded at different times (Khanna *et al.*, 1990, Anonymous, 1992-93).

Table 69. Effect or dam's body weight on birth weight.

Body weight of dam (kg)	Birth weight (kg)	Source
Upto 350	32.11 ± 1.70	Anonymous, 1992-93
351 - 400	35.54 ± 5.08	
401 - 450	36.59 ± 5.59	
451 - 500	38.63 ± 4.99	
501 and higher	39.83 ± 5.23	
Upto 500	31.1 ± 1.73	Khanna *et al.*, 1990
551 - 600	36.5 ± 1.24	
601 - 650	37.2 ± 1.53	
651 - 700	38.8 ± 0.98	
701 - 750	39.8 ± 1.10	
751. - 800	42.3 ± 1.21	
801 and higher	40.4 ± 1.54	

9. Effect of sire on birth weight.

The sire also influences birth weight in camels and mean difference in birth weight of Bikaneri camels has been observed to be as high as 6.83 kg due to sire effect (Barhat and Chowdhary, 1980). Effect of sires on birth weight of Bikaneri and Jaisalmeri camels has been summarised in Table 70.

Table 70. Effect of sire on birth weight.

Breed	Sire number	Birth wt. (kg)	Source
Bikaneri	16	45.64 ± 1.45	Barhat & Chowdhary, 1980
	89	43.36 ± 0.70	
	18	42.93 ± 0.60	
	101 A	42.60 ± 1.09	
	82	41.51 ± 1.09	
	07	39.32 ± 0.48	
	119	38.81 ± 1.26	
	85	38.38 ± 0.80	
Bikaneri	01	38.59 ± 1.94	Anonymous, 1992-93
	02	39.14 ± 1.99	
	03	40.61 ± 1.74	
Jaisalmeri	01	37.33 ± 2.40	
	02	38.00 ± 1.94	

10. Effect or stocking rate on birth weight in llama.

The only observation so far encountered in the available literatures has shown significant effect of stocking rate of llamas on pasture on the birth weight of cries of the virgin females (Table 71). The difference in birth weight due to stocking rate substantially reduced during the second parity (Vorano and Bertoni, 1984).

Table 71. Effect of stocking rate on birth weight.

Animals per ha of grazing land	Average birth weight (kg)	
	First year	Second year
0.5	6.90	8.5
1.0	5.85	8.0
2.0	5.70	8.6
Mean 1.17	6.15	8.37

Growth pattern in dromedary camels

Growth pattern measured as body weight gain has been observed in different breeds of Indian dromedary reared under variable management (Beniwal and Chowdhary, 1983, Chowdhary, 1986, Khanna *et al.*, 1990, Anonymous, 1992-93). The pattern of change in body weight with the progressive age has been found to be influenced by several factors like feeding and management, sex and breed of the camels (Table 72).

Average daily gain in body weight determined at 3 months interval from birth to 24 month of age, in the Bikaneri, Jaisalmeri and Kutchi breeds of Indian camels shows distinct effect of high milk suckling upto 6 months of age in all the breeds (Table 73). The rate of body weight gain has been found high upto 15 month of age which may be considered the period of active growth in the Indian breeds. A sharp fall in body weight gain during 9-12 month of age was probably due to significant reduction in the availability of milk associated with scarcity of browse as also may be seen during 15-18 month of age in Bikaneri and 18-21 month of age in Jaisalmeri and Kutchi camels (Anonymous, 1992-93).

Table 72. The pattern of change in body weight of Indian camels with progressive age.

Factors	Mean body weight (kg) at different age											
	Birth	3 m	6 m	9 m	12 m	1.5 yr	2 yr	2.5 yr	3 yr	5 yr	10 yr	15 yr
Bikaneri[1]	42.5	-	163.0	-	211.5	251.5	283.0	336.7	-	-	-	-
Do, male[2]	42.0	-	149.0	-	226.5	-	-	-	-	540.0	678.0	769.0
female	40.0	-	149.0	-	226.0	-	-	-	-	493.0	533.0	540.0
Bikaneri[3]	40.5	107.7	174.4	-	238.6	-	318.6	-	405.1	-	-	-
Kutchi[3]	34.0	96.4	157.8	-	207.4	-	262.5	-	361.3	-	-	-
Jaisalmeri[3]	28.8	94.7	135.4	-	181.7	-	265.0	-	320.0	-	-	-
Crossbred[3]	37.5	104.0	173.0	-	229.6	-	320.0	-	427.0	-	-	-
Bikaneri[4]												
Sire-1	39.1	100.4	143.7	159.9	172.1	-	-	-	-	-	-	-
Sire-2	38.6	92.6	144.1	167.4	191.9	-	-	-	-	-	-	-
Sire-3	40.6	110.1	152.5	164.0	176.3	-	-	-	-	-	-	-
Jaisalmeri[4]												
Sire-1	38.0	88.8	123.6	141.2	148.7	-	-	-	-	-	-	-
Sire-2	37.3	102.7	154.0	165.0	178.3	-	-	-	-	-	-	-
Kutchhi[4]	31.3	100.0	122.0	139.5	154.0	-	-	-	-	-	-	-

Sources: 1- Beniwal & Chaudhry, 1983; 2- Chowdhary, 1986; 3- Khanna *et al.*, 1990; 4- Anonyms, 1992-93.

Table 73. Mean daily body weight gain (g) in different breeds of camels at quarterly interval upto 24 month of age.

Age in month	Bikaneri	Jaisalmeri	Kutchi
Birth - 3	612.2 ± 17.3	571.8 ± 40.8	604.9 ± 38.8
3 - 6	650.5 ± 19.7	631.0 ± 32.8	582.7 ± 25.8
6 - 9	378.6 ± 39.2	382.5 ± 28.6	288.3 ± 26.2
9 - 12	303.0 ± 39.5	195.0 ± 37.4	182.0 ± 16.3
12 - 15	352.0 ± 21.6	313.1 ± 47.6	251.8 ± 32.7
15 - 18	220.3 ± 15.3	188.38 ± 31.4	175.6 ± 21.6
18 - 21	273.2 ± 26.5	127.7 ± 37.6	113.3 ± 21.6
21 - 24	268.4 ± 31.7	219.3 ± 40.7	196.7 ± 17.8

In another study also effect of milk availability of body weight gain patter is quite significant. The rate of gain is very high upto 6 month of age and selection for still higher growth rate is possible for veal production at 3 to 6 month of age in the Indian camels (Table 74). Distinct decline in growth rate has been observed at 6 and 12 months of age (Khanna *et al.,* 1990).

Table 74. Body weight gain pattern in Indian camels (g/day).

Age in month	Bikaneri	Kutchi	Arabian X Bikaneri
Birth - 3	732	800	749
3–6	616	686	664
6–12	349	254	373
12–24	209	132	207

The effect of birth weight on body weight gain has been found to be similar for most of the birth weight classes except the calves below 30 kg and higher than 50 kg birth weight gained at a lower rate (Table 75). The effect of environment is rather more than the effect of birth weight (Sahni *et al.,* 1992-93).

Table 75. Effect of birth weight on body weight gain (kg).

Birth weight (kg)		Body weight gain (kg)		
Range	Mean	0- 3 month	3 - 6 month	Total gain
Below 30	27.65 + 1.45	60.29 + 14.21	112.41 + 15.96	172.70
31 - 35	33.15 + 0.28	70.88 + 2.62	120.76 + 4.57	191.64
36 - 40	38.32 + 0.15	67.82 + 2.34	120.80 + 3.03	188.62
41 - 45	42.62 + 0.21	68.06 + 3.36	123.00 + 4.72	191.78
46 - 50	47.87 + 0.49	65.60 + 4.05	119.33 + 4.09	184.93
Above 50	53.33 + 0.88	57.33 + 7.45	110.00 + 11.7	167.33

High gain in body weight of camel calves has been also observed on the feeding of milk or milk substitute alongwith concentrate mixture and leguminus fodder. Dromedary calves gained at the rate of 750, 700 and 363 g per day from birth to 1 month suckling, 1-2 months on milk substitute feeding and 2-6 month on the feeding of normal diets respectively (Elias *et al.,* 1986). Still higher body weight gain has been observed on the feeding of whole milk after separation from the dam, which was 867 g upto 30 days of age and rose to 1 kg daily during 90-100 days of age. Average dally gain in body weight upto 180 days of age was 680 g (Degan *et al.,* 1987). Average body weight of the pure bred and crossbred dromedaries of Kazakastan has been found to be 310 and 413 kg respectively at 15 months of age (Aueljbekov, 1967).

Growth pattern in bactrian camels

The birth weight of bactrian camel is mostly in the range of 30 to 40 (mean 35) kg. In the countries of central Asia (earlier USSR) both bactrian and dromedary and their hybrids are reared. The calves are normally weaned at 8-10 month of suckling. Average body weight of bactrian, dromedary, bactrian X dromedary and dromedary X bactrian hybrid camels has been found to be about 87.6, 7.6, 87.2 and 104.0 kg respectively under otherwise similar management (Blagovescenskii, 1963) A significant difference in the male and female bactrian camel of Mongolia has been reported (Table 76). The males grew faster and attain higher body weight than the females at puberty and maturity (Panasenko and Luvsan, 1971). The Kazakh breed of bactrian camel is larger than the Mongolian bactrian and smaller than the Kalmykh breed. Averages daily gain in body weight ranges from 1268g to 2520g on good pasture during the wet-hot season in Kazakhastan (Dzhumagulov, 1982).

Table 76. Mean change in body weight of Mongolian bactrian camels of two sexes with progressive age.

Box	Number	Mean body weight (kg) at different age				
		Birth	6.5 m	1.5 yr	4.5 yr	7.5 yr
Male	15	35.9	129.0	250.1	481.0	611.3
Female	15	34.8	133.1	247.0	456.0	481.7

Growth pattern in new world cameloids/llmoids

Of the four species of cameloids, the llama and guanaco are largest and comparable in body size, whereas vicuna is smallest and alpaca stands in between (Cardozo, 1954 French, 1966). Average birth weight of llama is about 9.7 ± 0.1 kg, which becomes 53.9 ± 2.17 kg on weaning at about 223 days of suckling on ranges. Average daily gain in body weight during pre-weaning growth has been found to be 180 ± 5 g (Rodriguez and Torres-Hernandez. 1982). Average birth weight of alpaca is about 8 kg which is doubled in two months suckling giving about 133 g daily gain in body weight. At 3 years of age, average body weight of males is about 75 kg and that of the females is about 65 kg (Fernandez-Baca, 1975). The weaning has short duration adverse effect on the growth of young alpaca. An average 83 g daily gain in body weight recorded 12 days before weaning reduced to almost zero during the first 7 days post weaning and then again rose to about 110 g daily during the next 9 days. In another group, about 110 g daily gain 30 days before weaning fell down to zero gain during 8 days post-weaning but rose to about 37 g during the next 8 days (Pollard *et al.*, 1993).

The body weight and measurements of adult llamoids (Table 77) shows large variation (French, 1966).

Table 77. Body weight and measurements of llamoids.

Species	Body weight (kg)	Height (cm)	Length (cm)
Llama	90-110	100-125	100-131
Guanacoe	80-90	100-113	100-122
Alpaca	75-85	85-98	76-85
Vicuna	35-50	70-91	82-91

References

Anonymous, 1992-93. Annual report, National Research Centre on camel, Jorbir, Bikaner.

Aueljbekov, K. 1967. Camel breeding – a profitable field. Konevod. Konnyi Sport, 5: 6.

Barhat, N.K. and Chowdhary, M.S. 1980. Note of the inheritance of birth weight in Bikaneri camel (Camelus dromedarius). Indian J. Anim. Sci., 50: 665.

Barhat, N.K., Chowdhary, M.S. and Gupta, B.K. 1979. Note on relationship among gestation length, birth weight, placenta weight and intra-uterine development index in Bikaneri camel. Indian J. Anim. Res., 13: 115.

Beniwal, B.K. and Chaudhry, A.L. 1983. Growth pattern in Bikaneri camel (Camelus dromedarius). Indian J. Anim. Sci., 53: 101.

Bhargava, K.K., Sharma, V.D. and Singh, M. 1963. A study of the birth weight and body measurements of camels (Camelus dromedarius). Indian J. Vet. Sci. Anim. Husb., 35: 358.

Blagovescenskii, V. 1963. Reserves in the production of milk and meat. Konevod. Konnyi Sport, 33(10): 8.

Burgemeister, R. 1975. Elevage de chameaux en Afrique du Nord, 86 pp. GTZ, Eschborn.

Cardozo, Gonzales A. 1954. the auchenidae. La Paz., Bolivia. Chapman, M.J. 1985. Mongolia: Bactrian camel. World Anim. Rev., No. 55: 14.

Chowdhary, B. 1986. Some important biological and production characters of the Bikaneri camel. Indian J. Anim. Prod. Manage., 2: 145.

Degan, A.A., Elias, E. and Kam, M. 1987. A preliminary report on the energy intake and growth rate of early weaned camel (Camelus dromedarius) calves. Anim. Prod., 45: 301.

Dzhumagulov, I.K. 1983. Hybridization in camel breeding. Zhivotnovodstvo No. 9: 46.

Elias, E., Cohen, D. and Steimetz, E. 1986. A preliminary note on the use of milk substitute in the early weaning of Dromedary camel. Com. Biochem. Physiol., 85A: 117.

Fernandez-Baca, S. 1975. Alpaca raising in the high Andes. World Anim. Rev. No. 14: 1.

French, M.H. 1966. The Auchenidae. World Rev. Anim. Prod., 2(3):89.

Khanna, N.D., Tandon, S.N. and Rai, A.K. 1990. Breeding parameters of Indian camels. Indian J. Anim. Sci., 60: 1347.

Panasenko, A.G. and Luvsan, B. 1971. Age changes in live weight of Mongolian camels. Vest, Sel'-khoz. Nauki, Alma-Ata, 14(4): 59.

Pollard, J.C., Littlejohn, R.P. and Davis, G.H. 1993. Changes in live weight and behaviour of alpaca dams and offspring following weaning. New Zealand Vet. J., 41: 161.

Rodriguez, C.T. and Torres-Hernandez, G. 1982. A genetic study of some production traits in the llama (Lama glama) on the high plateau in Bolivia. 1. Meat production. Memdoria, Assoc. Latinoamericana de Prod. Anim., 17: 35.

Terentjev, S.M. 1951. Experience in stud work on a camel breeding farm. Konevodstvo, 11: 20.

Vorano, A.E. and Bertoni, J.A. 1984. Biological and production traits of llamas (Lama glama, Cuvier) on natural pasture with supplementation of different stocking rates. Revista Argentina de Prod. Anim., 4: 325.

□□□

Chapter 7

Meat and Meat Products

All species of camelidae are sacrificed for the production edible meat for human consumption but there is large variation in meat characteristics and these are considerably influenced by the kind of animals slaughtered for meat production. The conditions of the animals are largely dependent on the supply of feeds and water. In wet season, availability of nutritious fodders increases and condition of animals improves. Thus, carcass yield is higher. In some of the pastoral societies of Africa, the camels are rarely slaughtered for meat production and camel meat is a luxury, while in some other African countries a large number of camels mostly spent and culled one are slaughtered for human consumption locally and in the neighbouring countries. Camel meat production is well-organised in Ethiopia, Kenya, Somalia and Sudan and in these countries, camels are most reared for meat export to other countries (Leupold, 1968, Williamson and Payne, 1973). In Libya, Saudi Arabia and other gulf countries, large number of finished camels are imported for slaughter from Ethiopia, Kenya, Sudan and other countries.

The consumption of meat is generally more in cold countries and bactrian, dromedary and their crossbreds are slaughtered in large number in different countries of central Asia, Mongolia and China (Terentjev, 1963, Kulaeva, 1964, Cerenpuncag and Davaa, 1967, Zhang *et al.*, 1983). The small size New World cameloids of the South America are mainly reared in large flocks on high lands for the production of good quality fibres and meat (Tapia Cano, 1965, Fernandez-Baca, 1975).

Due to fast development in modern methods of transport, the utility of the camels as working animal is diminishing at a rapid rate in many countries but the demand of meat is increasing, which has opened newer avenue for the rearing of camels for meat production. In some countries of central Asia and China, the hybridization between the bactrian and dromedary species is quite popular for increasing the production of meat and milk (Aueljbekov, 1967).

In some nomadic groups the camel blood is also used as a food item for human consumption. Besides using the blood collected at slaughter, the camels are also bled periodically in some pastoralist groups and the frequency of bleeding may be upto twice a month (Pratt and Gwynne, 1977).

Camel Veal

Since the utility of male camels as pack and riding beast is decreasing at a fast rate, the males and surplus female calves may be reared for the production of good quality veal. Milk yield of both bactrian and dromedary camels is quite high and even after full feeding of calves, considerable amount is spared for human consumption.

A high rate of body weight gain in suckling calves of both bactrian and dromedary camels have been recorded in early life. The body weight at birth is almost doubled in about two and half month of suckling in the Mongolian bactrian calves (Chapman, 1985). The rate of daily gain in body weight of the Bikaneri, Kutchhi and crossbred camel calves during first three months of suckling period is an average 732, 800 and 749 g daily (Khanna *et al.*, 1990). The rate of growth may be also influenced by other factors and in a subsequent report, the average daily gain in the body weight of the Bikaneri, Jaisalmeri and Kutchhi camel claves during the first three month of life has been 612, 572 and 605 g respectively (Anonymous, 1992-93). The hybrids of dromedary X bactrian exceed the body weight gain by 20 per cent of the mid-parent value (Dzhumagulov, 1983). Mean body weight of bactrian, dromedary, bactrian male X female dromedary and dromedary male X bactrian female at the end of three months suckling has been recorded aboat 87.6, 79.6, 89.2 and 104.0 kg respectively (Blagovescenskii, 1963). The body weight at birth, 6-8 kg in alpaca and llama is doubled in about two months of suckling. Average daily gain in the body weight of Arabian camel calves is about 870 g during the first month of life against 8 liters milk intake per kg gain in body weight (Degan *et al.*, 1987). The camel calves weaned at the end of 30 days suckling can be successfully reared on the feeding at a good quality milk substitute. An average 780 g daily gain in the body weight has been observed on the ding of milk substitute during the second month (Elias *et al.*, 1986).

Camel meat

A good quality meat is produced from the slaughter of young camels below 3 years of age and it is relatively more economical to slaughter at about 2.5 years of age because bactrian calves gain at the rate of 26 kg per year from weaning at 12-18 months age to 2.5 years of age and after this annual body weight gain declines to about 10 kg in arid zone of Kazakhstan (Ahmediev, 1966). However, in most of the countries called animals are largely slaughtered for meat production. The lean carcass of dromedary contains very little fat which is generally higher in aged (more then 5 years of age) animals and females (Nasr *et al.*, 1965). The meat of spent bactrian is generally inferior than the well-finished younger animals (Cerepuncag, 1969).

Method of Slaughter

In most of the countries, usual halal method is followed for the slaughter of the camels. The animals are secured with its head extended in a definite direction depending on the place of slaughter. The slaughter starts from the ventral surface at the point of the larynx and blood vessels including the trachea and oesophagus are cut quickly with the help of a sharp knife.

The nerves and vertebrae are left intact and bleeding is allowed. Some modification has been made in the slaughter method in south Darfur. The animal is restrained couched with the longitudinal axis of the body pointing to Mecca and the animal is stabbed in the heart with a sharp knife. The head is cut off immediately and hide is separated from the dorsal line securing the animal still in the couched position (Wilson, 1978).

Body weight of different species at slaughter

Average body weight at slaughter is generally heavy for the bactrian camels than the dromedary camels. The body weight of South American camelids is much less being 5-10 per cent the bactrian and dromedary camels (Table 78).

The nerves are left intact and bleeding is allowed. A little modification has been made in the slaughter method in South Darfur. The animal is restrained couched with the longitudinal axis of the body pointing to Mecca and the animal is stabbed in the heart. The head is cut off immediately and hide is separated from the dorsal line securing the animal still in the couched posture (Wilson, 1978).

Table 78. Body weight of the camels and camelloids at slaughter.

Species/Type	Country	Sex	Body weight (kg)	Source
Bactrian	China	Male	646.3	Zhang *et al.*,1983
		Female	529.9	
	Russia	Male	438.0	Dzhumagulev, 1982
	Russia	Male	700 – 850	Terentjev, 1963
		Female	450 - 500	
	Mongolia	Male	630	Cerenpuncag and
		Female	497	Davaa, 1967
Dromedary	Somali	Male	554	Congiu, 1953
		Female	514	
	Sudan	Male	448	Wilson, 1978
	Female	414		
Alpaca	Peru	Male	57 – 72	Tapia Cano, 1965
		Female	50 – 66	
	3 years	Male	75	Calderon and
		Female	65	Fernandez Baca, 1972
Llama		84		Rodriguez and Torres Hernandez, 1982
Vicunna		35 – 40		Fernandez Baca, 1975

Carcass characteristics

Carcass yield and Dressing percentage

The carcass yield depends on the body condition of the animals at slaughter and it is influenced by the species, type, breed, age, sex, level of feeding and management. The bactrian camels are generally heavier than most of the dromedary breeds. The different species of lama are much smaller in comparison to one-humped and two-humped camels. The values of carcass yield and dressing percentage in relation to various factors have been summarised in Table 79. Carcass yield and dressing percentage values are generally high in males than the females (Cangiu,1953, Wilson, 1978, Zhang *et al.,* 1983). These values are also higher in younger than the spent aged animals (Kuleava, 1964, Sohail, 1983). Dressed carcass also includes hump, kidneys and kidney fat but not other edible organs (Wilson, 1978).

The mean carcass weight 208.5 + 38.78 (SD) kg contains about 120.2 + 22.21 kg fore quarter, 84.5 + 14.53 kg hind quarter and 4.0 + 4.30 kg hump, which constitute about 57.65, 40.53 and 1.92 per cent of the dressed carcass and about 35.0, 24.7 and 1.1 per cent of the slaughter weight respectively in the dromedary camels of Sudan (Wilson, 1978). In addition about 17 kg empty stomach and intestines and other edible organs are also produced.

Table 79. Carcaa yield and dressing percentage in relation to various factors in different species.

Species/Type	Age/Grade	Sex	Body weight (kg)	Carcass wt. (kg.)	dressing (%)	Source
1	2	3	4	5	6	7
Bactrian	Adult	Male	700-850		56-63.3	Terentjev, 1963.
		Female	450-500		do	
	2 yr 8 m				62.8	Kulaeva, 1964
	19-20 yr				55.9	
	Adult	Male	630	338.9	53.8	Cerenpuncag and
		Female	497	267.4		Davaa, 1967
	Grade I		480	249	51.9	Cerenpugcag, 1969
	Grade II		422	207	49.1	
	Grade III (spent)		445	212	47.6	
		Castrate	646.3	359.6	55.6	Zhang *et al.*, 1983
		Female	529.9	255.5	48.2	
		Castrate	750-850	375-425	50.0	Chapman, 1985
Dromedary	Adult	Male	554	310.8	56.1	Congiu, 1953
		Female	514	278.1	54.1	
		Male	447.9	231.3	51.4	Wilson, 1978
		Female	414.4	196.3	47.4	

	Adult		660	381.1	57.74	Babiker, 1984
	32 m	Male				62.79 Sohail, 1983
	32 m	Female			55.80	
	10-12 yr	Male			56.14	
	10-12 yr	Female			54.14	
Alpaca	Adult	Male	66.8	32.3	48.00	Tapia Cano, 1965
		Female	58.6	30.5	52.00	
	3 yr	Male	75	45	60.00	Caderon and
		Female	65	35.75	55.00	Fernandez Baca, 1972

Grading of Carcass

So far probably there is no international standard grading system for the camel carcasses. Generally, carcasses in retail markets are classified as the carcass of young animals, carcass of well-finished animals and carcass of spent and aged animals. The carcass of young animals is light pink in colour and contains more moisture and little fat. The carcass of good finished camels is pinkish in colour and contains moderate distribution of fat besides considerable amount of depo fat. The ratio of fat mainly depends on the plane of nutrition. The carcass of spent old animals is dark coloured and coarse with various degree of fattyness depending on the plane of nutrition and sex. These animal are mostly 12-20 years old females culled after the production of 6 - 8 calves and also the aged males retired from drought uses. Some information available on the grading of carcasses are highly variable. In some centrel Asian countries (old USSR), the carcasses with medium fat deposition are first grade, high fat deposition are second grade and the carcasses of old camels are third grad. (Table 81). The last grade contains very little fat in most.of the cases but very high bone percentage (Kuznetsov and Tret'yakov, 1970). Contrary to this in Mongolia, lean meat with low moisture and high fat percentage is first grade, with medium moisture and medium fat content is second grade and that containing high moisture and low fat (Table 80) and obtained from aged animals is third grade (Cerepuncag, 1969).

Table 80. Dissectable tissue percentage in carcass.

Species	Grade	Lean	Fat	Bone	Source
Bactrian		82.0		18.0	Dzhumagulov, 1982
do		75.0	8.8	16.2	Zhang *et al.*,, 1983
Dromedary	I	76.6	4.8	15.9	Kuznetsov and
	II	67.6	6.8	21.4	Tret'yakov, 1970
	III	52.8	0.0	38.1	

Composition of the dissectible tissues in the carcass

The percentage of dissectible tissues viz, lean meat, fat and bones depends on the finishing of the carcass (Table 81). Bones in the carcass constitute about 15.9 to 38.1 per cent of the total carcass weight and it is very high with little fat in the carcasses of aged and spent camels (Kuzmetsov and Tret'yakov, 1970, Dzhumagulov, 1982, Zhang *et al.*,

1983). Average carcass length .of female bactrian of China is 167.7 cm with 60.3 cm^2 eye muscle area and in females the corresponding values are 157 cm and 49.4 cm^2 (Zhang *et al.,* 1983).

Chemical composition of lean mean

The chemical composition of lean meat of the camels varies with age at slaughter (Nasr *et al.,* 1965) and carcass grade (Cerepuncag, 1969). The most variable component in camel carcass like other ruminant carcass is fat content (Table 81). The fat percentage is always high in the muscles of the sternal region.and it is higher in females then in the males. High fat content in the perinoporic than the hump meat is invariably found (Nasr *et al.,* 1965).

Table 81. Chemica1 composition of meat (%)

Carcass	Grade/age	Moisture	Protein	Fat	Ash	Source
Bactrian	Grade I	58.86 - 61.49	17.41 - 18.46	20.12 - 22.84	0.81 - 0.92	Cerepuncag, 1969
	Grade II	63.75 - 70.18	18.30 - 19.48	9.30 - 17.00	0.95- 1.01	
	Grade III	69.71 - 74.89	19.10 - 21.30	2.74 - 10.63	0.96- 1.07	
Dromedary -						
below 5 yrs age		78.27	20.07	0.92	0.76	Nasr *et al.,* 1965
above 5 yrs age		76.24	22.02	1.01	0.86	

*Fat dissected lean meat.

Yield of offals and hide

The range and average yield of liver, heart and lungs, skinned head, skinned feet and hide is present in Table 82. The stomach and intestines constitute about 5 per cent of the body weight and these are used for the preparation of casings for the manufacture of stuffed meat products like sausage, etc. The main waste material is gut fill which is an average 75 kg in adult males and abut 88 kg in adult females constituting about 16.8 and 21.3 per cent of the body weight respectively (Wilson, 1978). The gut contents are the main source of pollution in the abbateir. From large abbateirs, it is collected for the preparation of organic manure and in small abbateirs it creates cleaning problem.

Table 82. Yield of offals and hide.

Offals	Weight (kg)		Per cont of body wt.	
	Range	Mean	Range	Mean
Liver	4.5 - 11.0	7.5	1.47 - 3.45	2.8
Heart lungs	6.5 - 10.5	8.4	1.78 - 3.36	2.5
Skinned head	8.5 - 16.5	12.1	2.80 - 4.49	3.6
Skinned feet	10.5 - 19.5	14.6	3.31 - 5.16	4.3
Raw hide	22.5 - 47.0	34.8	8.50 - 11.76	10.2

Meat of Cameloids

The meat of all cameloids is used as human food and that of young alpaca and vicuna is considered more delicious than the meat of the adult animals. Since the cria (lambs) of different species of the New World cameloids are generally slaughtered for the production of pelt, the tender meat (veal) is available for human consumption. A considerable number of animals below one year of age are also slaughtered for meat production. The meat of such animals is also delicious and more acceptable because it does not omit the characteristic odour normally emitted from the meat of the adult animals. The meat of adult alpaca resembles mutton but omits strong characteristic odour which persists even after cooking. For economic and other reason, the animals are preferably slaughtered at about 3 years of age when average body weight of the males is about 75 kg and that if the females is about 65 kg and carcass yield is about 60 and 55 per cent respectively (Calderon and Fernandez Baca, 1972). In most of the flocks, about 8 per cent aged animal and infertile females are also culled and killed for meat production.

References

Ahmediev, A. 1966. The meat production of camels. Konevod. Konnyi Sport, 36(2): 12.

Annonymous 1992-93. Annual report of the National Research Centre of Camel. Indian Council of Agricultural Research, Bikaner.

Aueljbekov, K. 1967. Camel breeding – a profitable field. Konevod. Konnyi Sport, 5: 6.

Babiker, M.M. 1984. Abundance and economic potential of camel in the Sudan. J. Arid Environ., 7: 377.

Blagovescenskii, V. 1963. Reserves in the production of milk and meat. Konevod. Konnyi Sport, 33(10): 8.

Calderon and Fernandez Baca, S. 1972.

Cerepuncag, S. 1969. Meat productivity of camels. Konevodstvo No. 10:34.

Cerepuncag, S. and Davaa, R. 1967. Camel breeding in Mongolia. Mezhdumar Sel'khoz. Zhurmal, 11(3): 107.

Chapman, M.J. 1985. Mongolia : Bactrian camels. World Animal Rev. No. 55: 14.

Congiu, S. 1953. Dressing percentage, weight distribution and correlation between different parts of the body in Somali dromedary. Zootec. e Vet., 8: 188.

Degan, A.A., Elias, E. and Kam, M. 1987. A preliminary report on the energy intake and growth rate of early weaned camel (Camelus dromedarius) calves. Anim. Prod., 45: 301.

Dzhumagubov, I.K. 1982. Selection and breeding of Kazakh camels. Dairy Sci. Abstr., 46: 652 (Abstr. 5734).

Dzhumagubov, I.K. 1983. Hybridization in camel breeding. Zhivotnovodstve No. 9: 46.

Elias, E., Cohen, D. and Steimetz, E. 1986. A preliminary note on the use of milk substitute in the early weaning of dromedary camels. Comp. Biochem. Physiol., 85A: 117.

Ferenandez Baca, S. 1975. Alpaca raising in the high Andes. World Animal Rev., No. 14: 1.

Khanna, N.D., Tandon, S.N. and Rai, A.K. 1990. Breeding parameters of Indian camels. Indian J. Anim. Sci., 60: 1347.

Kuleava, V. 1964. The production of the bactrian camel. Konevod. Konnyi. Sport, 34: 9.

Kuznetsov, V.A. and Tret'yakov, V.N. 1970. Carcass classification in Turkman single-humped camel. Trudy Turkmen, Sel'khoz. Inst., 15: 130.

Leupold, J. 1968. The camel : Important domestic animal of Sub-Tropic. In: Les cahiers bleus veterinaries, 15: 1.

Nasr, S., El-Bahay, G. and Moursy, A.W. 1965. Studies on camel meat. 1. The effect of age and sex on the components of camel meat. J. Arab. Vet. Med. Assoc., 25: 253.

Pratt, D.J. and Gwymme, M.D. (Eds) 1977. Rangeland management and Ecology in East Africa. Hodder and Stoughton, London.

Rodriguez, C.T. and Torres-Hernandez, G. 1982. A genetic study of some productive traits in the llama (Lama glama) on the high plateau in Bolivia. 1. Meat productions. Memoria Assoc. Latiniamericana de Prod. Auch., 17: 35.

Sohail, M.A. 1983. The role of the Arabian camel (Camelus dromedarius) in Animal production. World Rev. Anim. Prod., 19: 37.

Tapia Cane, C. 1965. Production of alpaca meat. Vida agric., 42: 499.

Terentjev, S.M. 1963. Camel breeding in Astarkhan Province. Zivetnovodstvo, 25(1): 54.

Williamson, G. and Payne, W.J.A. (Eds.) 1978. An introduction to Animal husbandry in the Tropics. 3rd edn., Longman, London.

Wilson, R.T. 1978. Studies on the livestock ed southern Darfur, Sudan. V. Notes on camels. Trop. Anim. Hlth. Prod., 10: 19.

Zhang, P.Y., Zuo, Z.T., Zhao, H. and Bai, G.H. 1983. Carcass evaluations of bactrian camel. Chinese J. Anim. Sci., 1: 29.

❑❑❑

Chapter 8

Fibre Production

The two-humped bactrian camel of the cold deserts and the cameloids (llamoids) of the high altitude of South America produce fairly large quantity of good quality wool fibre. The yield of fibre from the dromedary of hot desert is very low. The fibres obtained from different camelids are generally soft, light durable. The heat conductivity of camelids hair is very low due to which it is extensively used for the manufacture of woollen fabrics and garments. The fleece of alpaca with shorting fibre is similar to the fleece of Corriedale sheep (Fernandez-Baca, 1975). Of the four llamoid species, the lammas are reared for wool production and work and alpaca and vicuna for wool production. The guancoe are killed for hide and flesh (Cardozo, 1954). A considerable decrease in the fibre yield of bactrian camels from an average 3.4 kg in 1929 to less than 1.7 kg has been obtained at some farms of the old soviet provinces in 1982 (Bairamov and Gavrichkin, 1983). This is believed to be the sequalae of the removal of camels from ranges to intensive rearing at the organised farms.

Fibre Yield

Being the beast of hot desert, fibre production of single-humped dromedary camel is very low and in most of the animals, 1-2 kg annual clip is obtained. However, the dromedaries in cold climates also produce upto 5 kg fleece during clipping in the spring season (Nanda, 1957, Singh, 1966, Sohail, 1983). Annual hair yield from bactrian camels is 4-7 kg but in some cases, it may be 12-16 kg (Terentjev, 1953). Some heavy males and castrates of Mongolian bactrian have yielded upto 18 and 10 kg per annum respectively (Chapman, 1985). Non-pregnant females produce about 25 per cent more fibre than the lactating females and quality of wool is better from the pure bred camels than the crossbreds (Kulaeva, 1964). However, hybrids produce more wool than the mid-parent production value (Dzhumagulov, 1983).

Earlier the llamoids were primarily reared for the production of wool and pelt, but subsequently meat production also gained importance. Wool production from the llama and alpaca is 2.5-5.0 kg under good management, and from vicuna 0.25-0.6 kg (Chivilchez Chavez, 1959, Duga, 1986). However, there is large variation due to several factors like age, sex, stocking rate, castration and culling intensity. In llamoid flocks with low culling rate, annual fleece yield is less than 1.38 kg (Rodriguez and Torres-Hernandez, 1982, Vorano and Bertoni, 1984). The yield of fibres from the camels and llamoids has been summarised in Tables 83 and 84.

Table 83. Yield of fibre per clip from the camels.

Species/	Male	Castrate	Female	Average	Source
Dromedary	-	-	-	1.5-2.0	Sohail, 1983
Do	-	-	-	4.0-5.0	Singh, 1966
Bactrian					
Kazakh	-	-	-	4.5	Podberezkin, 1951
Astarkhan	12	-	6	5.7-6.3	Terentjev, 1963, 1963
Kalmykh	9	-	5.7		Terentjev, 1966
Kalmykh	-	-	4.0-5.5		Kulaeva, 1964
Mongolian	6.5	-	5.0		Cerenpuncag and Davaa, 1967
Mongolian	18	10	-	5.0	Chapman, 1985
Bactrian				6.8	Dzhumagulov, 1983
Dromedary				2.6	
Hybrids				5.2	

Table 84. Wool yield from different llamoid species.

Species	Wool (kg)	Source
Alpaca	1.8 (1-4)	Fernandez-Baca, 1975
Llama	1.3	Rodriguez & Torres-hernandez, 1982
Llama, 1st year-	2nd yr.	Vorano & Bertoni, 1984
2 per ha	1.24 -1.28	
1 per ha	1.25 -1.35	
0.5 per ha	1.32 -1.38	
Alpaca	3.62	Chivilchez Chavez, 1956
Llama	2.78	
Vicuna	0.59	
Alpaca	1.5 - 5.0	French, 1966

Huancoe	1.0 - 2.0	
Llama	1.5 - 3.5	
Vicuna	0.18 - 0.32	
Alpaca	3 - 5	Duga, 1986
Guanaco	0.5	
Llama	2.5 - 3.7	
Vicuna	0.25	

Characteristics of camel hair

Although hair is clipped from both the species, the yield from dromedaries of hot desert is 1-2 kg but from those migrated to cold areas, it may be 4-5 kg. The fibre of dromedary is largely used for the preparation of rugs and ropes by the cameliers themselves. The bactrian camel contributes significantly in wool production. The wool is soft, light and durable and has low heat conductivity. Best quality wool is produced by the yearlings with more than 85 per cent non-medullated fibres of 16-18 um diameter against the coarser clips of adults containing higher percentage of medullated fibres and 76-83 per cent clean wool (Terentjev, 1963).

Rough hairy wool is obtained from the mane, knees, chest and elbow region, which constitute about 15-30 per cent of total fleece (Terentjev, 1963, Luvsan, 1969, Chapman, 1985).

The site of wool collection has significant influence on the quality. Clean wool yield from the flank region is 79.1-92.6 per cent against 78.3-87.5 per cent in the neck wool besides differences in other traits (Table 85). The colour of wool from the Kalmyk type of bactrian camel is white to dark brown and that of Mongolian is reddish. The wool colour varies from white to reddish in the crossbreds (Potokina *et al.,*, 1991). The cost colour of dromedary is mostly light (pale) brown to dark brown but white and black coated animals are also found.

Table 85. Yield of clean wool and fineness of fibres of bactrian camels.

Types of bactrian	Clean wood yield (%)		Fineness of fibre (um)	
	Flank	Mane	Flank	Mane
Adult Kalmyk male	84.5	47.6	26.40	38.60
Adult Kalmyk female	73.4	50.0	27.32	31.02
Yearling Kalmyk	75.9	67.0	22.44	24.36
Adult Mongolian	72.6	38.6	22.41	34.30
Kalmyk X Mongolian	82.6	-	24.32	-

The coarse (hard) wool obtained from the knees, chest, elbow and name of the total fleece production. The length of fibre is 69-334 mm and diameter is 46-74 um. The 1ength of the fine wool fibres from the sides of the neck, body and legs is 50-157 and diameter is 21-29 um (Chapman, 1985).

Characteristics of llamoid wool

There is wide variation in the colour, length and fineness of the fibre between different llamoid species. The fibre of llama is coarse and its colour ranges from white to black. White wool is preferred but pelts of all colour had good demand. The 'Chaku' type llama is more woolly than the 'Ccara' type. The coat colour of alpaca shows similar variation as in llama but fibre is finer. The alpaca fibre is graded 80' on the Bradford scale against 60' for the wool of Merino sheep (Hugh-Jones and Bacon, 1964). The staple of 'Suri' type alpaca is long and straight and resembles with the wool of Lincoln sheep. The fibre of 'Huacaya' type alpaca is short and curly as found in Corridale sheep. The coat colour of guanaco is mostly reddish brown or light brown (French, 1966). The fibre of guanaco has low value but the demand of pelt is of young animals is very high. The coat colour of vicuna varies from pale yellow through vermilion and golden to fulvous (Dennler De La Tour, 1954). Wool fibre of vicuna is extremely fine and it is graded 120-130' on the Bradford scale (Koford, 1957). A bib of long and coarse hairs hangs from the brisket of the vicuna. The colour of bib and abdominal fibres is white as seen in Blackbuck (Antelope cervicapra). The crosses between the alpaca and vicuna are most wanted due to higher yield of fine fibre than the yield from vicuna (Fernandez-Baca, 1975). Some information on fibre traits have been summarised in Table 86.

The wool and pelt of llamoids have high commercial value and used for the preparation of good quality garments and fancy items. Pelt of aborted full term foetuses is specially collected for the preparation of ladies purse and baby coats.

Table 86. Fibre traits of llamoids.

Species	Clean wool (%)	Fibre length (cm)	Diameter (um)	Medullation (%)	Kemp hair (%)	Source
Alpaca	83	39	25.25	-	-	A
Llama	82	26	30.78	-	-	A
Vicuna	79	10	14.24	-	-	A
Guanaco	-	-	13.83	5.4	1.9	B
Llama	-	-	19.68	13.5	1.2	B
Vicuna	-	-	13.44	3.8	1.1	B
Alpaca	-	10-30	15-40	-	-	C
Guanaco	-	10-15	50-100	-	-	C
Llama	25-30	30-120	-	-	C	
Vicuna	-	4-8	10-12	-	-	C
Llama	-	3.34 + 0.68	53.19 + 1.39	-	-	D

Sources : A = Chivilches Chavez (1956);
B = Utkular *et al.* (1963); C = French (1966);
D = Rodriguez arid Torres-Hernandez (1982).

Hides and Skins

The commercial value of camel hide is low due to lower yield of good quality 1eather (Wilson, 1984). The yield of hide varies with the age, sex and size of the animal and it is generally 27-39 kg per adult animal (Terentjev, 1963).

The furred skin and pelt of the llamoids are valuable by-products due to their larger use for the production of fancy goods.

References

Bairamov, D. and Gavrichkin, V. 1983. Camels should be returned to the desert. Konevod. Konnyi Sport, 7: 11.

Cardozo, Gonzales A. 1954. The auchenidae. La Paz., Bolivia.

Cerenpuncag, S. and Davaa, R. 1967. Camel breeding in Mongolia. Mezhdunar Sel'khoz. Zh., 11: 107.

Chapman, M.J. 1985. Mongolia : Bactrian camels. World Animal Rev., No. 55: 14.

Chivilichez Chavez, J. 1956. Structure and management of the wool of the llama family (alpaca, llama and vicuna). Rev. Patron. Biol. Anim. (Madr.), 2: 355.

Denneler De La Tour, G. 1954. The vicuna. Oryx, 2: 347.

Duga, L. 1986. The most important characters of fibres from South American camelidae (llama, alpaca and their crosses and guanacos). Lanas, Seminario Cientifico Tecnico Regional, 3 de Setimber a l de Octobre de, 1985.

Dzhumagulov, I.K. 1983. Hybridization in camel breeding. Zhivotnovodztvo No. 9: 46.

Fernandez-Baca, S. 1975. Alpaca raising in the high Andes. World Animal Rev. No. 14: 1.

French, M.H. 1966. The Auchenidae. World Rev. Anim. Prod. 2(3):89.

Hugh-Jones, M.E. and Bacon, A.J. 1964. The 'Augenidos' of South America. The Veterinarian, Oxford, 2: 251.

Koford, C.B. 1957. The vicuna and the puna. Ecol. Monogr. 27: 153.

Kulaeva, V. 1964. The production of the bactrian camel. Konevod. Konnyi Sport, 34: 9.

Luvsan, B. 1969. Some economic and biological traits of Mongolian two-humped camels. Zh. Zhivot. Vet. (1972), 2: 58.

Nanda, P.N. 1957. Camels and their management. 17 pp. Indian Council of Agricultural Research, New Delhi.

Podberezkin, Ja. 1951. Experience of the work of a better camel breeding farm. Konevod. Konnyi Sport, 10: 42.

Potokina, L.I., Tsyrendondokov, N.D. and Al'Baev, I. 1991. Basic wool traits of bactrian camels of different genotypes at the "Akgaraiskii" breeding farm. Anim. Breed. Abst., 1994, 62: 74.

Rodriguez, C.T. and Torres-Hernandez, G. 1982. A genetic study of some production traits in the llama (Lama glama) on the high plateau in Bolivia. 2. Wool production. Memoria, Assoc. Latino Americana de Prod. Anim., 17: 45.

Singh, H. 1966. Camel care. Intensiv Agric., January, p. 9.

Sohial, M.A. 1983. The role of the Arabian camel (Camelus dromedarius) in animal production. World Rev. Anim. Prod., 19(3): 37.

Terentjev, S. 1953. Work of the Astarkhan state breeding co-operative breeding and perfecting the Astarkhan breed of camels. Konevod. Konnyi Sport, 23: 20.

Terentjev, S.M. 1963. Camel breeding in Astrakhan province. Zivotnovodstvo, 25: 54.

Terentjev, S. 1966. Improvement of the Kalmyk breed of camel. Konevod. Konnyi Sport, 36: 19.

Utkanlar, N., Imeryuz, F., Oznacar, K. and Muftuoglu, S. 1963. Studies on the fitness and colour characteristics of the Turkish hairy goat wool and their comparison with those of cashmere, llama, vicuna and guanaco wools. Lalahan Zootek. Arast. Enst. Derg., 3(2): 8.

Vorano, A.E. and Bertoni, J.A. 1984. Biological and production parameters in the llama (Lamag lama, Cuvier) on natural pastures of the high Andean plateau, with supplementation and different stocking rates. Rev. Argentina de Prod. Anim., 4: 325.

Wilson, R.T. 1984. The camel. Longman, London.

Chapter 9

Camels for Draught

Inspite of considerable progress in modern power driven transport facilities, the utility of camels as the draught animal power is still important for the sandy soils of deserts and riverines in many countries including India. The dromedary camels are normally classified as the riding camels of slender body, light weight and active habits and baggage camels of large size, heavy built and slow pace (Hira, 1947, Islamy, 1950, Iwema, 1960). Similarly, bactrian camels are also the beast of burden in the cold deserts of central and East Asian countries (Terentjev, 1963, Cerenpuncag and Davaa, 1967). The camels are used to perform different kinds of work like carrying of pack load, ploughing of arable land, pulling of cart and persian wheel and local oil pressing machines, etc. (Wilson, 1978, Khanna and Rai, 1994).

The Riding Camels

The riding camels are selective bred for light frame, slender body and long legs. These are normally thin animals with slender and compact body, long and strong limbs, smooth leg bones and strong foot hold. The adult riding bull camels should have masculine disposition, boldness, alertness and symmetry. The face is generally short with high domed forehead, short and triangular ears and prominent eyes. Somewhat flattened roman nose, deep muzzle and even lips are the other features. The neck is slender, short, muscular which evenly blends with the shoulder at the base. The shoulders are deep, strong and well-covered. The ventral aspect from chest to posterior half or two-fifth is almost straight and then deeply concave due to sudden bending. The neck should be held in an inverted 'L' shape with poll at the level of the hump. The ribs should be wide and well sprung with elbow carried clear from the lower part of the chest. The muscles of chest and arms should be strong. The back is short, hump is well-formed and even, loins smooth and rump is moderately dropping. The things are broad, thick and full. Similar should be the built of the part immediately below (gaskin or second thigh). Hamstring should be strong and elastic. The forearms should be muscular with strong and heavy knee joints. The hock joints should be moderately straight and flexible. The common and sannon bones should be clean and flat. The front feets are fairly straights, whereas rear feets are slightly turned out. The soles show even wear in the camels of plain but uneven in the hilly camels. The skin should be thin and supple and covered with smooth short hairs.

The feets of riding camels are like the pneumatic rubber tyres in which air has been replaced by the pads of fatty tissue. The fat is deposited in a series of pads separated by the cartilaginous septae and enclosed by a strong wall of collagenous fibres except at the posterior end, where elastin is the main component. The fatty pads are formed of neutral triglycerides containing about three-fourth unsaturated fatty acids. The fat pad is fairly liquid even in cold climate due to which movement of the camel is not hampered even during the winter season and also in cold deserts. The fatty pads are enclosed in a thick rubbery epidermis which is constantly moistened by the secretion of sweat glands in the epidermis (Bligh *et al.*, 1976) The venous blood from the solar corium is drained by the branches of the abaxial and axial proper digital veins. The solar corium has very rich plexuses, which are represented by a single layer formed by the veins of different sizes. (Osman *et al.*, 1987).

Performance of the riding camels

A riding camel carrying a single rider with approximately 54 kg baggage may run at the rate of 10 km per hour and may cover 45-50 km distance in 4-5 hours (Dina and Klintegerg, 1977). On the other hand, a camel carrying only single rider may run 15-20 km per hour and can cover about 80 km daily (Leese, 1927). Indian riding camels are normally driven 60-80 km daily in the deserts of Thar (Matharu, 1966).

There is no uniformity in the description of pace of the riding camels. Four different speeds have been described by Leese (1927) but he has given about 4, 3-12 and 14-19 km hourly speed for walk, jog and fast run respectively, and no speed has been mentioned for canter. Islamy has given a range of 6-24 km per hour without differentiation for the riding camels of Iran-shahr (1950). Two speeds i.e., the slow trot of about 8 km per hour and fast run of 16-32 km per hour have been given for the male 'Beja' and 'Anafi' camels of Sudan (Gillespis, 1962). For the Indian riding camels three speeds viz., (3-5 per hour), jog (8 km per hour) and canter or fast run (13-15 km per hour) have been suggested (Matharu, 1966). The canter or fast run pace is hardly maintained for an hour and this exercise is exhaustive for both, the beast and the rider. Alternate names for these speeds are walk. Trot and gallop or center (Cauvet, 1925). The fast run, gallop and canter are used as synonyms in camels, whereas in race horses walk, trot, canter and gallop indicate progressive increase in speed as well as the mode of running.

Training of the riding camels

Initially young camels are driven with the use of nosepeg, nose-ring, bridle or halter in different countries. These devices are normally applied in early age below 2 years. The training for smooth development of running speeds normally starts at about 3 years of age (Singh, 1963, Matharu, 1966). Delay in training often results in stubborn and unruly behaviour (Nanda, 1957, Knoess, 1976). The training of riding camels starts with the obedience teaching consisting of head control, which is achieved by the characteristic movement of the rope tied with nose-peg or otherwise and vocal command of the trainer or rider. This is followed by teaching for sitting and rising on command, and to allow smooth mounting in the sitting posture (Leese, 1927).

The training for changing speed starts with walk and during this period, the animal is taught to respond to the movement and tension of the reins. After this the camels are trained for different speeds. A riding camel should never be struck on the back of his neck and if necessary, it should be tickled behind the right leg of the rider (Singh, 1963) and should be trained to respond to the kicks of different intensity by the rider on the abdomen of the animal.

Baggage/ Draught camels

The camels used for carrying pack loads, pulling carts, persian wheel for irrigation, oil pressing and ploughing are mostly slow paced animals of heavy built. The baggage camels are generally large and heavy with heavy bones suitably covered with muscles. The animal with roman nose, prominent eyes, large lips and well-formed head are preferably selected for draught purposes (Acland, 1932). A medium to long neck with head held high and deep chest with well-formed last ribs are the desired traits. The back should be longer to hold a baggage saddle. The straight forelimbs should be wide apart and these should not be turned outwards. Such formation causes brushing at the elbow. The bones of limbs should be heavy and strong and feets should be large and flat.

Performance of draught camels

The camels are most suitable beast of burden for the sandy soil of hot deserts and can carry loads for 25-30 km in 6-8 hours walking (Matharu, 1966). A pack load of 150-300 kg can be carried for 6-8 hours but heavy load (450 kg) can be carried to a short distance only. The Bikaneri camels used regularly carry about 200 kg baggage for 6-8 hours (Sharma and Bhargava, 1963). Heavy animals may carry 250-300 kg load for 30-50 km daily (Hira, 1947). Riverine type camels are frequently used to haul merchandise (200-300 kg per trip) in two rounds upto a distance of 10 km and only one to and fro round, when distance covered is beyond 10 km. About 1-3 hours rest is given to the camel after each trip and some feed is offered during the resting hours.

The draught camels can be worked on metalled roads also and a pair of Indian camels can pull 1.5-2.0 tonnes load on a two or four wheel cart for a distance of 30-40 km in about 4 hours time provided the tyres are pneumatic and wheels are fitted with bell bearings. About 90-125 kg draught force is generated by a camel and it is 17-22 per cent of body weight. The draught camels are able to plough at a pace of about 2.5 km in an hour and about 500 m^2 land can be ploughed per hour (Khanna and Rai, 1994). The camels should not be worked for more than 6 hours in a stretch and more than 8 hours a day (Singh, 1966).

Training of draught camels

The training of draught camels for carrying pack load or pulling carts, etc. starts at about 2 years of age. In third year light loads are carried and from fourth year animals may be used regularly (Iwema, 1960). In India, training begins at 3 to 4 year of age depending on the condition of the animal and maximum performance is achieved at about 8 years of age (Hira, 1947).

Different types of baggage saddles are used in different countries but all are fitted with soft pads for protecting the skin from bruising.

The materiel to be pack loaded is divided into two equal halves and loaded by balance to hang on either side of the hump. Sometimes, a third bag is loaded accross the basal bags over the hump. In such cases, the two side bags are fixed at a higher level on either side to avoid unwanted pressure on the hump. Camels should never be driven on clay or mud during the rains, otherwise it may be disastrous. Camels once fallen frequently break their bones and perhaps never recover to perfect working condition.

Use of llamoids for riding and work

Among the four species of llamoids of South America, only llamas and guancoes are used for riding and carrying pack loads on the high hills. The hybrids of llama and alpaca are very bad pack animals. The llamas, preferably the males are used for riding and carrying a load of 25-35 kg depending on the distance to be travelled and also the terrain to be covered. The llamas do not carry heavy loads and and on forced loading sit down. It responds only when load is reduced to his carrying capacity. These are very notorious animals and do not hesitate spitting on the face of the rider, when tired (Fernandez-Baca, 1975).

Production of dung energy

The camelids void faeces in the shape of pellets which normally contains less than 50 per cent moisture. The faecal pellets are used as fuel and manure.

References

Acland, P.B.E. 1932. Notes on the camel in eastern Sudan. Sudan Notes Rec., 15: 119.

Bligh, J., Thomson, J.L.C. and MacDonald, A.G. 1976. Surface contact structures. In: Environmental physiology of animals. Blackwell Publications, Oxford, U.K.

Cauvet, C. 1925. Le Chemeau. J.B. Billiere et fils, Paris.

Cerenpuncag, S. and Davaa, R. 1967. Camel breeding in Mongolia. Mezhudunar Sel'khoz. Zh., 11: 107.

Dina, D. and Klintegerg, R. 1977. Proposal for a rural development training project and study concerned with camel utilization in arid lands in Ethiopia. Mimeo, Relief and Rehabilation Commission, Addis Ababa.

Fernandez-Baca, S. 1975. Alpaca raising in the high Andes. World Animal Rev., 14: 1.

Gillespie, I.A. 1962. Riding camels of the Sudan. Sudan J. Vet. Sci. Anim. Husb., 3: 37.

Hira, L.M. 1947. Camel breeding in Indian. Indian Farming, 8: 504.

Islamy, A. 1950. Riding camels around Khas and Iranshahr. Rev. Fac. Med. Vet., Tehran, 12: 87.

Ivwema, S. 1960. The ship of the desert. Veeteelt. en Zuivelbe-richtan, 3: 390.

Khanna, N.D. and Rai, A.K. 1994. In Arid Regions - Use of camel as draft animal should be encouraged. Indian Farming, 44(3): 23.

Knoess, K.H. 1977. The camle as a meat and milk animal. World Animal Rev., 22: 139.

Leese, A.S. 1927. A treatise on the one-humped camel in health and disease. Haynes and sons, Stamford.

Matharu, B.S. 1966. Animal management: Camel care. Indian Farming, 16(7): 19.

Nanda, P.N. 1957. Camels and their management. 17 pp. Indian Council of Agricultural Research, New Delhi.

Osman, F.A., Arnautovic, I. and El-Khaligi, G.M. 1987. Venous drainage of the corium and other structures of the foot of one-humped camel (Camelus dromedarius). Assiut Vet. Med. J., 18(36): 1.

Sharma, V.D. and Bhargava, K.K. 1963. The Bikaneri camel. Indian vet. J., 40: 639.

Singh, H. 1963. Handbook of animal husbandry for extension workers. Ministry of food and Agriculture, Directorate of Extension, Krishi Bhavan, New Delhi.

Singh, H. 1966. Camel care. Intensive Agric., January, p. 9.

Terentjev, S.M. 1963. Camel breeding in Astrakhan province. Zivotnovodstvo, 25: 54.

Wilson, R.T. 1976. Studies on the livestock of southern Darfur, Sudan. 5. Notes on camels. Tropical Anim. Hlth. Prod., 10: 10.

□□□

Chapter 10

Behaviour and Management of the Camel

Behaviour of the One-humped Camel (*Camelus dromedarius*)

The general behaviour and attitude of the one-humped camel have been observed closely and compiled to provide useful information for the handling and management (Singh, 1966). The characteristic behaviour of dromaderies has been listed as follows :

1. The camel although decile, should not be believed particularly the musth males. They are highly vindictive by nature and do not forget rude and unkind treatment for long time. Whenever such camels get a chance, they attack the person and may bite or even kill him for unkind treatment like beating and scolding.

2. Male camels may not be aggressive only to strangers but even to his own attendant during the rutting season. Rutting male exhibit radical changes in behaviour. It becomes aggressive, often unapproachable and bites, if gets chance (Yagil and Etzoin, 1980).

3. The camels are slow and sluggish in nature, but they may have remarkable power of indurance and would work till death without showing any apparent sign of fatigue. Hence, it is for the attendant to know the behavioural changes due to fatigue in his camel.

4. The camels are generally unmindful when spoken to or patted, but they respond then called with a handful of green fodders or grains.

5. Normally a healthy camel sits in an upright and straight posture with raised head. Any sideways inclination of the body with head held low and the neck often laid down on the ground may be regarded as the signs of illness and should be attended accordingly.

6. The camel frequently opens it mouth and emits gurgling and bellowing sounds. A person unfamiliar with such habits of the camels may get frightened.
7. Faecal pellets and urine are passed frequently in small amounts at a time. Urine is normally splashed with tail on the back parts of the body. This is for facilitating body heat loss through evaporation of urine from the body surface.
8. The camel is a good swimmer but does not like to enter in the water unless compelled.
9. They prefer browsing on tail trees and shrubs but they can also graze on herb and grasses, when browse is not available. The camels are capable to feed on thorny plants due to special structure of lips, oral papillae and oral secretion.
10. The camels are capable to live without water for several days in hot season and for weeks in cold season. They can easily tolerate upto 30 per cent dehydration. Dehydration is required within short time after drinking water.
11. Breeding in camel is seasonal and mating takes place in sitting posture, both mates facing in the same direction.
12. Musth male does not tolerate any rival. Other junior and weaker males suppress their sexual desire due to fear of the rutting male. However, such males can exhibit rut on separation and herding with the females.
13. The female in oestrus likes the company of males specially the musth one and frequently presses and pushes the non-rutting males to stimulate their sexual activities.
14. Lactating female ceases to eject milk on weaning her calf. A few may adopt a foster calf. Use of skin of a dead calf on the body of another calf or the dummy calf from the skin of dead calf may stimulate milk ejection. Inflicting pain by beating to forget the calf has also helped in some cases.

Normal values of Temperature

Respiration rate and Pulse (Heart) rate in camelids

The rectal temperature is normally elevated by 2-3°C in the afternoon. The elevation in temperature occurs due to work, excitement and irritation. Perspiration in dromedary camels start when rectal temperature exceeds 40.5°C (Higgins and Kock, 1984). Dromedary camels may tolerate considerable rise in body temperature and fluctuation upto 7°C has been observed in dehydrated camels (Schmidt-Nielsen *et al.*, 1981). The rise in body temperature is a normal phenomenon in the camel exposed to heat and dehydration and it does not cause metabolic disturbances upto certain extent. Llamoid, guanaco is still higher tolerant to ration as elevation in body temperature is only 0.5°C in dehydrated guanac (Mofarlane, 1964) • The dromedary is capable to decrease metabolism for reducing internal heat production on dehydration and direct exposure to the sun (Yagil *et al.*,1978). The body coat is an excellent insulating material and provides protection to camels both, against cold as well as heat Mcfarlane, 1964). Under normal conditions the body coat sheds off in the summer but it is retained in deficient supply of drinking water or otherwise water deprivation for longer period during the hot season (Yagil *et al.*, 1974).

All camelid species are covered with dense coat during the winter season (Bustinza, 1979).

Respiration and pulse rates also rise in the evening (Bhatt *et al.*, 1960), Higgins and Kock, 1984). Some information available on body temperature, respiration rate and heart rate are presented in Table 87.

Table 87. Mean values of temperature, respiration and heart rate of different camelids.

Species	Particulars	Rectal °F	temperature °C	Respiration rate per minute	Heart rate per minute	Source
Dromedary (Indian)	Morning, Minimum	95.2	35.1	5	25	Bhatt *et al.*, 1960
	Maximum	99.7	37.6	10	44	
	Average	97.9	36.6	7.5	33	
	Evening, Minimum	98.5	36.9	6	30	
	Maximum	101.7	38.7	11	48	
	Average	100.0	37.8	9	36	
(Arabian)	Morning	96.8-97.7	36-36.5	5-10	30-45	Higgins & Kock, 1984
	Evening	102.2	39.0	12	35-50	

Rectal temperature in llamoids Bligh *et al.*, 1975

		At sea level °F	°C	At high altitude °F	°C	°F	°C
Alpaca	Minimum	100.2	37.9	99.7	37.6	-	-
	Maximum	100.9	38.3	100.8	38.2	-	-
Llama	Minimum	100.6	38.1	99.0	37.2	-	-
	Maximum	101.5	38.6	100.4	38.0	-	-
Vicuna	Minimum	-	-	96.8	36.0	99.3	37.4
	Maximum	-	-	100.2	37.9	102.4	39.1

Camel management practices in the Indian subcontinent

The various management practices of camel husbandry followed by the cameliars of the Indian subcontinent have been recorded carefully. These include grooming, clipping, oiling and mud smearing (Nanda, 1966). Mud smearing is not followed on the organised farms.

Grooming : The objectives of grooming the camels are to keep the animals clean and healthy by removing dirt and foreign bodies, eliminating ectoparasites like ticks and mites and stimulating peripheral blood circulation. Grooming also provides an opportunity to detect injuries, parasites, abscess and other external defects, if any. Grooming is easier in hot season when body coat is short, but it becomes tidious in winter due to long end slaggy body coat. A stable (dandy) brush of hair bristles, thatch or plastic and a curry comb are used for the grooming of the animals. The curry comb is held in left hand with its dentine upwards and stable or body brush in the right hand. Grooming of camels starts from the base of the ears in the direction of hairs and carried through neck, shoulder, chest, hump, body, belly, thigh and ends at the tail. This is followed by the grooming of limbs including the brisket region. The eyes, nostrils, armpits, groin and genital organs are cleaned with a damp piece of clean cloth. A piece of clean gunny bag or rug is also used far the grooming of camels. In case of long outdoor journey, a handful of dry long grass free from injurious foreign matters may also be used for the grooming of the animals.

Clipping : The camels are normally clipped after winter in the spring season which is normally March-April in the Indian subcontinent. Hand sheers or clipping machines used for horses are used for the clipping of camels. The animals are clipped close to body surface and in baggage camels the saddle region is left unclipped as a preventive measure against the formation of gall due to continuous friction by the saddle on the back. Clipped camels may need protection from cold, if temperature is still low. This is provided by covering the animal with a 'Jhul' or housing in a shed during the night.

Oiling : After clipping the animals, rape seed oil or mustard oil is applied thoroughly all over the body. This makes the skin glazy and also protects from direct exposure to environment. Being mud irritant, oiling also stimulates peripheral blood circulation.

Mud smearing : After about 48 hours of oiling the camel is taken to a clean mud hole for smearing a reasonably thick layer (1.5 - 2 cm thick) of clay mud on the body of the clipped camel. The mud layer is left undisturbed on the body for three days and then removed by stripping off. Mud smearing after clipping is used for providing protection from the bites of insects and infestation of ectoparastes and other dermal infections.

Housing : The camels are herded in open during night in the hot season and in daytime, they rest under the trees while browsing. However, at the organised farms and stall feeding, the camels are housed in well ventilated sheds made of thatch, asbastos sheets or concrete. Tall and shade providing trees should be planted around the camel sheds for providing protection from solar radiation and hot wind. Sheds should be constructed in a direction to provide protection frog the direct wind. The males, females and young animals should be housed in separate sheds. Rutting males are tied secured in individual shed for avoiding fight causing injury to other males.

Salt feeding : Crushed rock salt should be offered to camels at the rate of 45-60 g daily or 135-180 g. at three days interval, mixed in farm grains mixture. Composite minerals mixtures used for cattle may also be used for the camels. Salt feeding is very important, as most of the fodders eaten by the camels contain inadequate amount of sodium chloride. Craving for salt is often noticed in herds, where salt feeding is casual and occassional.

Watering : The camel is capable to live without water for considerable time due to which it survived and prolifereted in deserts whether hot or cold desert . The ability to bear water deprivation is affected by several factors like atmospheric temperature, humidity and wind movement, age, sex and breed and the type of work done by the animal, and water content of herbages eaten. The camel should normally be offered water for drinking at 3-7 days internal in hot season (about 40°C), at 2-3 weeks interval when temperature is moderate (25-30°C) and occassionlly in cold season. However, it should not be over exploited. Water deprived dromedaries may consume upto 135 litres in less than 15 minutes time and camels derive 3-30 litres water daily from the browse (Gauthier-Pilters, 1974). Daily water requirement of Indian camels is 14-36 litres but in deprived animals, it may be upto 91 litres (Leese, 1927).

Feeding : Normally camels are allowed 6-8 hours browsing daily, which may decrease to total stall feeding, when used for working for several hours. The diets of stall fed animals may contain green forages hay, straw and concentrate mixture with a handful of common salt. Wheat straw mixed with concentrate mixture and moistened with water in the form of 'sani' is normally fed to riverine type Indian camel. They are fed tree leaves of pipal, neem, pakar and bamboo leaves besides several kinds of herbs and cultivated fodders.

Milking : The camels are milked twice daily in morning and evening, but it some countries more frequent milking at 6-8 hours interval is also practiced. The camels are milked in standing position. Sometimes fastening of hind limbs with a rope may be necessary for restraining an unruly female.

Restraints used for controlling camels

Appliances used for restraining the camels differ in different countries. In Indian subcontinent, use of metallic nose peg or halter is more common. Nose ring and bridle are also used for driving the camels. Nosepegs of wood and bone are used in some Arabian and African countries. A nosepeg or nose ring of about 2-3 cm diameter is pierced preferably in the left nostril at a young age of less than two years (Singh, 1963). Occasionally both nostrils are pierced specially for controlling the unruly camels. Training of camels after 3 years of age often becomes troublesome (Nanda, 1953).

Riding camels should not be struck on the back of their neck. For increasing the speed, it is better to strike gently on the abdomen behind the right leg of the rider (Singh, 1963).

Health management

Some preventive measures may be essential for maintaining healthy herds. Preventive measures depend on the types of health problems prevalent in an area. Generally deworming of young calves, prevention or both infestation and mange are the common practices. Preventive vaccination against some viral and bactrial diseases may be necessary in endemic areas.

Disposal of dung

The dung is hard peletted and does not produce problem of disposal in healthy herds. The dung pellets are stored either in open exposed to sun drying for use as fuel or in a pit along with other farm wastes for composting for manure. The frequency of defaecation and amount of daily dry matter void in faeces depend on the level of feeding. About 350-500 g faecal dry matter is voided per 100 kg body weight (Schmidt-Nielsen *et al.*, 1956, Matharu, 1966, Maloiy, 1972).

References

Bhatt, P.L., Kohli, R.N. and Rathore, U.S. 1960. The normal body temperature, respiration frequency and heart rate of the camel. Indian vet. J., 37: 456.

Bligh, J., Baumann, I., Sumar, J. and Pacco, F. 1975. Studies of body temperature pattern in South American Camelidae. Comp. Biochem. Physiol. A, 50: 701.

Bustinza, A.V. 1979. South American camelids. Proc. IFS Intern. Symp. on camels, Sudan, pp. 73-108.

Gauthier-Pilter, H. 1974. The behaviour and ecology of camels in Sahara with special reference to nomadism and water management. Proc. Symp. on the behaviour of Ungulates and its relation to management, Calgary, p. 542.

Higgins, A.J. and Kock, R.A. 1984. A guide to the clinical examination, chemical restraint and medication of the camel. British Vet. J., 140: 485.

Leese, A.S. 1927. A treatise on the one-humped camel in health and disease. Haynes and sons, Stamford.

Maloiy, G.M.O. 1972. Comparative studies on the digestion and fermentation rate in the fore-stomach of the one-humped camel and zebu steer. Res. Vet. Sci., 13: 476.

Matharu, B.S. 1966. Animal management: Camel care. Indian Farming, 16(7): 19.

Mcfarlane, W.V. 1964. Terrestrial animals in dry heat: ungulates. Pp. 509-539 in Handbook of Physiology (Ed. Dill). American Physiological Society, Washington.

Nanda, P.N. 1957. Camels and their management. Indian Council of Agricultural Research, New Delhi.

Nanda, P.N. 1966. Management of camels. Indian Farming, 15(12): 38.

Schmidt-Nielsen, B., Schmidt-Nielsen, K., Houpt, T.R. and Jarnum, S.A. 1956. The water balance of the camel. American J. Physiol., 185: 185.

Schmidt-Nielsen, K., Crawford, E.C. and Hammael, H.T. 1981. Respiratory water loss in camels. Proc. Royal Society, London, 211: 291.

Singh, H. 1963. Handbook of Animal Husbandry for Extension Worker. Ministry of Food and Agriculture, New Delhi.

Singh, H. 1966. Camel care. Intensive Agric. Jan. p. 9.

Yagil, R. and Etzion, Z. 1980. Hormonal and behavioural patterns in the male camel. J. Reprod. Fertil., 58: 61.

Yagil, R. Sod-Moriah, U.A. and Meyerstein, N. 1974. Dehydration and camel blood. American J. Physiol., 226: 298.

Yagil, R., Etzion, Z. and Ganani, J. 1978. Camel thyroid metabolism: Effect of dehydration. J. Appl. Physiol., 45: 450.

□□□

Subject Index

A

Arabian camel 4
Auchenidae 4
Alpaca 4
Abomasum 59
Accessory sex glands 93
Age at first service 110
Age at first conception 116
Alternate mating system 122

B

Bactrian camel 4
Behaviour 215
Blood 23
Blood composition 23
Blood definition 23
Blood functions 24
Blood physical properties 24
Blood cells 27
Blood plasma 27
Blood serum 27
Blood volume 26
Blood cell membrane 32
Blood inorganic constituents 45
Blood sugar 45
Buccal cavity 54
Blood plasma 39
Blood plasma composition 39
Breeding 87
Breeding season 128
Butter 166
Birth weight 177
Body weight at birth 177
Body weight effect of species 177
Body weight at breed 178
Body weight at lactation 178
Body weight at cross breeding 178
Body weight at hybridization 178
Body weight at sex of calf 179
Body weight at parity 179
Body weight at calving month 180
Body weight at dam weight 180
Body weight at sire 181
Body weight at stocking rate 182
Behaviour of camel 215
Baggage camels 211
Bactrian camel 4

C

Camelids of modern era 3
Camelloids 3
Camels nomanclature 2
Camels bactrianus 4
Camels dromedory 4
Camelus bactrianus 4
Camelus dromadarus 4

Camelids, zoological classification 8
Camel breeding purpse 8
Camelids socio-economic importance 9
Camel-a ship of desert 11
Camel world distribution 11
Complex chambged stomach system 56
Compartment C1 57
Camel calf rearing 78
Cervix 107
Calving interval 118
Calving rate 120
Coitus 133
Copulation duration 134
Colostrum 151
Cream 168
Cheese making 169
Camel veal 190 (Camveal)
Camel meat 191 (Camflesh)
Carcass yield 192
Carcass cutting 195
Carcass composition 195
Chemical composition of lean meat 196
Camel management 219
Courtship in camels 132
Courtship in llamoids 133
Critical haematological values 31

D

Dromedary camel 4
Draught power of camelids 17
Digestion 53
Digestive system 53
Dental formula 55
Digstive system functions 64
Digestion end products-fate 67
Digesta passage 70
Digestion of feeds 76
Ductus deferens 90
Double hump camel 129
Dromadory camel 131, 145
Dressing percentage 192
Dung production 213
Draught camel 209, 211
Draught camel performance 212
Draught camel training 213
Dung disposal 221
Dromadom female 131

E

Erythrocyte 27
Erythrocyte count 29
Erythrocyte dimension 28
Erythrocyte sedimentation rate 29
Erythrocyte count 29
Erythrocyte fate 31
Erythrocyte life span 31
Epididymis 89

F

Fibre production 16, 201
Fibre of camelids 18
Faveolar epithelium 62
Feeding behaviour 67
Feed selection on rangeland 68
First calving age service age 110
Female reproductive system 103
Fertility rate 120
First conception age 116
Foetal fluids 126
Foetal membranes 126
Fermented milk products 169

Fibre yield 201
Fibre characteristics 203

G

Glandular mucosa of stomach 60
gland isthmus epithelium 61
Gland endpiece epithelium 61
Gestation length 117
Growth in camelids 177
Ghee 168
Growth pattern in bacterian camel 183
Growth pattern in dromadory camel 182
Gowth pattern in hybrid camels 184
Guanaco 5
Growth in camelids 177

H

Hide production 16, 205
Haematology 23
Haemostasis 26
Homaeostasis 26
Haemoglobin 33
Haematocrit 30
Heat 111
Hormonal changes deving pasturition 127
Health management 221

I

Incisors 55
Intestines 63
Inter calving period 118

K

Khoa 169

L

Lama glama 5
Lama guvancoe 5
Lama pacos 5
Lama vicugna 36
Llama 5
Llamoids 4
Leucocytes 35
Leucocytes characteristics 36
Leucocytes fate 38
Leucocytes functions 38
Life span of crythrocytes 31
Liver 63
Llamoids 131
Let down of milk 148
Lean meat 196

M

Management 215
Meat production 14
Milk production 14
Mean carpuscular volume 134
Mean carpuscular haemoglobin 134
MCVE 135
Mouth 54
Male reproductive system 87
Mammary glands 145
Mammary external structure 145
Mammary internal structure 145
Mammary involution 146
Milk 145
Milk composition 154
Milk products 145, 168
Milk of camelids 153
Milk physical properties 153
Milk antimicrobial property 154

Milk composition, factors affecting 154
Milk proteems 157
Milk lipids 159
Milk mineals 160
Milk vitamins 161
Milk yield 161
Milk eat down 149
Milk yield, factors affecting 165
Milk yield, effect of feed 165
Milk yield, effect of water restruction 165
Milk yield, effect of body weight 166
Milk yield, effect of season 165
Milk yield, effect of hybridization 167
Mawa 169
Meat 189
Meat products 189
Meat of camelids 197
Meat characteristics of llamoids 204
Management of camels 215
Mating 133
Membrane of blood cells 32

N

Nomenclature of camels 2
New homes of camelloids 12
Nitrogenous fractious of blood 40
Nutrition 53
Neonatal calf behaviour 128

O

Oesophagus 55
Ovulation 107
Ovaries 104
Oviduct 104

P

Production potential of camelids 13
Packed cells volume 30
PCV 30
Platelets 38
Plasma lipids 43
Pharynx 55
Pancreas 64
Penis 91
Penis protrusion 94
Primary spermatocytes 96
Post partum oestrus interval 115
Pregnancy duration 117
Pregnancy signs 122
Pseudopregnancy 122
Pasturition 123
Post pastum behaviour of matter 127
Pulse 216
Pyloric mucosa 63

R

Respiration 216
Restraint of camels 221
Red blood cells (RBC) 27
Red blood cells count 27
Red blood cells dimension 28
RBC sedimentation rate 29
Reticulum 58
Rumen 57
Rumen contents 75
Rumen microbiology 75
Riding camel 209
Riding camel performance 210
Riding camel training 211
Reproduction 87

S

Socio-economic importance of camglids 9
Serum protein fraction 31
Spleen 64
Serotum 87
Spermatogenesis 95, 102
Spermatozoa 95
Site of pregnancy 122
Services per conception 116
Seasonal behaviour of male 129
Seasonal behaviour of female 131
Seasonal behaviour of bactrian female 131
Seasonal behaviour of edromedary female 132
Slaughter method 191
Slaughter weight 191
Skin 205
Salivam glands 56

T

Temperament of dromadary 13
Thrombocytes 38
Thrombocytes functions 38
True stomach 59
Testes 88, 99
Teats of bactrian camel 148

U

Uterus 106
Udder 148

V

Vicuna 6
Vicugna vicugna 6
Voluntary feed intake 68
Vas deferens 90
Vagina 107
Vestibule 107
Vulva 107

W

World distribution of camels 11
White blood corpuscles 35
WBC 35
White blood cell 35

Z

Zoological classification of camelids 8

❑❑❑